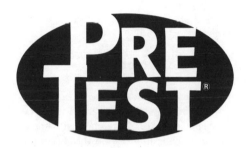

Medicine

PreTest® Self-Assessment and Review

Notice

Medicine is an ever-changing science. As new research and clinical experience broaden our knowledge, changes in treatment and drug therapy are required. The authors and the publisher of this work have checked with sources believed to be reliable in their efforts to provide information that is complete and generally in accord with the standards accepted at the time of publication. However, in view of the possibility of human error or changes in medical sciences, neither the authors nor the publisher nor any other party who has been involved in the preparation or publication of this work warrants that the information contained herein is in every respect accurate or complete, and they disclaim all responsibility for any errors or omissions or for the results obtained from use of the information contained in this work. Readers are encouraged to confirm the information contained herein with other sources. For example and in particular, readers are advised to check the product information sheet included in the package of each drug they plan to administer to be certain that the information contained in this work is accurate and that changes have not been made in the recommended dose or in the contraindications for administration. This recommendation is of particular importance in connection with new or infrequently used drugs.

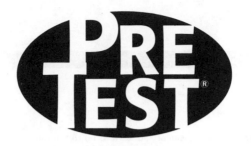

Medicine
PreTest® Self-Assessment and Review
Tenth Edition

Steven L. Berk, M.D.
Regional Dean
Professor of Medicine
Mirick-Myers Endowed Chair in Geriatric Medicine
Texas Tech University School of Medicine at Amarillo

William R. Davis, M.D.
Chairman and Associate Professor
Department of Internal Medicine
Texas Tech University School of Medicine at Amarillo

Robert S. Urban, M.D.
Associate Professor
Department of Internal Medicine
Texas Tech University School of Medicine at Amarillo

McGraw-Hill
Medical Publishing Division
New York   Chicago   San Francisco   Lisbon   London   Madrid   Mexico City
Milan   New Delhi   San Juan   Seoul   Singapore   Sydney   Toronto

Medicine: PreTest® Self-Assessment and Review, Tenth Edition

1 2 3 4 5 6 7 8 9 0   DOC/DOC   0 9 8 7 6 5 4 3

ISBN 0-07-140287-X

This book was set in Berkeley by North Market Street Graphics.
The editor was Catherine A. Johnson.
The production supervisor was Phil Galea.
Project management was provided by North Market Street Graphics.
The index was prepared by North Market Street Graphics.
RR Donnelley was printer and binder.

This book is printed on acid-free paper.

Library of Congress Cataloging-in-Publication Data

Medicine : PreTest self-assessment and review.—10th ed. / [editors] Steven L. Berk,
    William R. Davis, Robert S. Urban.
        p.; cm.
    Includes bibliographical references.
    ISBN 0-07-140287-X (alk. paper)
        1. Medicine—Examinations, questions, etc.   I. Berk, S. L. (Steven L.), 1949–
    II. Davis, William R., 1951–   III. Urban, Robert S.
    [DNLM: 1. Medicine—Examination Questions. W 18.2 M4914 2003]
    R834.5.M4 2003
    616'.0076—dc21   2003044246

Contributors

Misty Evans, M.D.
Assistant Professor of Medicine
Department of Internal Medicine
Texas Tech University School of Medicine at Amarillo

Marjorie Jenkins, M.D.
Assistant Professor of Medicine and Obstetrics & Gynecology
Department of Internal Medicine
Texas Tech University School of Medicine at Amarillo

Stephen P. Kelleher, M.D.
Associate Professor of Medicine
Department of Internal Medicine
Texas Tech University School of Medicine at Amarillo

Student Reviewers

Karen E. Groff
Robert Wood Johnson Medical School
Piscataway, New Jersey
Class of 2003

Sabari Nandi
Robert Wood Johnson Medical School
Piscataway, New Jersey
Class of 2003

Contents

Introduction . . . . **xi**
Acknowledgments . . . . **xiii**

Infectious Disease

Questions **1**
Answers, Explanations, and References **16**

Rheumatology

Questions **29**
Answers, Explanations, and References **38**

Pulmonary Disease

Questions **47**
Answers, Explanations, and References **60**

Cardiology

Questions **71**
Answers, Explanations, and References **90**

Endocrinology and Metabolic Disease

Questions **103**
Answers, Explanations, and References **116**

Gastroenterology

Questions **127**
Answers, Explanations, and References **137**

Nephrology

Questions **147**
Answers, Explanations, and References **157**

Hematology and Oncology

Questions 167
Answers, Explanations, and References 179

Neurology

Questions 195
Answers, Explanations, and References 204

Dermatology

Questions 215
Answers, Explanations, and References 223

General Medicine and Prevention

Questions 229
Answers, Explanations, and References 240

Allergy and Immunology

Questions 249
Answers, Explanations, and References 254

Geriatrics

Questions 259
Answers, Explanations, and References 263

Women's Health

Questions 267
Answers, Explanations, and References 275

Bibliography 281
Index 283

Introduction

Medicine: PreTest® Self-Assessment and Review, Tenth Edition, is intended to provide medical students, as well as house officers and physicians, with a convenient tool for assessing and improving their knowledge of medicine. The 500 questions in this book are similar in format and complexity to those included in Step 2 of the United States Medical Licensing Examination (USMLE). They may also be a useful study tool for Step 3.

Each question in this book has a corresponding answer, a reference to a text that provides background for the answer, and a short discussion of various issues raised by the question and its answer. A listing of references for the entire book follows the last chapter.

To simulate the time constraints imposed by the qualifying examinations for which this book is intended as a practice guide, the student or physician should allot about one minute for each question. After answering all questions in a chapter, as much time as necessary should be spent reviewing the explanations for each question at the end of the chapter. Attention should be given to all explanations, even if the examinee answered the question correctly. Those seeking more information on a subject should refer to the reference materials listed or to other standard texts in medicine.

Acknowledgments

We would like to offer special thanks to:

Our wives, Shirley Berk, Janet Davis, and Joan Urban, for moral support and helpful suggestions;

Our children, Jeremy Berk, Justin Berk, Abby Davis, Kyle Davis, David Urban, Elizabeth Urban, and Catherine Urban;

Our staff, Margie McAlister and Jackie Hammett, for excellent support in organizing, collating, and typing the manuscript;

Texas Tech University School of Medicine at Amarillo—in the pursuit of excellence;

Our previous student, Sheila Haffar, M.D., of Texas Tech University School of Medicine, for review of the text.

Infectious Disease

Questions

DIRECTIONS: Each item below contains a question or incomplete statement followed by suggested responses. Select the **one best** response to each question.

1. A 30-year-old male patient complains of fever and sore throat for several days. The patient presents to you today with additional complaints of hoarseness, difficulty breathing, and drooling. On examination, the patient is febrile and has inspiratory stridor. Which of the following is the best course of action?

a. Begin outpatient treatment with ampicillin
b. Culture throat for β-hemolytic streptococci
c. Admit to intensive care unit and obtain otolaryngology consultation
d. Schedule for chest x-ray

2. A 70-year-old patient with long-standing type 2 diabetes mellitus presents with complaints of pain in the left ear with purulent drainage. On physical exam, the patient is afebrile. The pinna of the left ear is tender, and the external auditory canal is swollen and edematous. The peripheral white blood cell count is normal. The organism most likely to grow from the purulent drainage is

a. *Pseudomonas aeruginosa*
b. *Staphylococcus aureus*
c. *Candida albicans*
d. *Haemophilus influenzae*
e. *Moraxella catarrhalis*

Items 3–4

A 25-year-old male student presents with the chief complaint of rash. There is no headache, fever, or myalgia. A slightly pruritic maculopapular rash is noted over the abdomen, trunk, palms of the hands, and soles of the feet. Inguinal, occipital, and cervical lymphadenopathy is also noted. Hypertrophic, flat, wartlike lesions are noted around the anal area. Laboratory studies show the following:

Hct: 40%
Hgb: 14 g/dL
WBC: 13,000/µL
Diff:
    Segmented neutrophils: 50%
    Lymphocytes: 50%

3. The most useful laboratory test in this patient is

a. Weil-Felix titer
b. Venereal Disease Research Laboratory (VDRL) test
c. Chlamydia titer
d. Blood cultures

4. The treatment of choice for this patient is

a. Penicillin
b. Ceftriaxone
c. Tetracycline
d. Interferon α
e. Erythromycin

Items 5–7

A 20-year-old female college student presents with a 5-day history of cough, low-grade fever (temperature 100°F), sore throat, and coryza. On exam, there is mild conjunctivitis and pharyngitis. Tympanic membranes are inflamed, and one bullous lesion is seen. Chest exam shows few basilar rales. Laboratory findings are as follows:

Hct: 38
WBC: 12,000/μL
Lymphocytes: 50%
Mean corpuscular volume (MCV): 83 nL
Reticulocytes: 3% of red cells
CXR: bilateral patchy lower lobe infiltrates

5. The sputum Gram stain is likely to show

a. Gram-positive diplococci
b. Tiny gram-negative coccobacilli
c. White blood cells without organisms
d. Acid-fast bacilli

6. This patient is likely to have

a. High titers of adenovirus
b. High titers of IgM cold agglutinins
c. A positive silver methenamine stain
d. A positive blood culture for *Streptococcus pneumoniae*

7. Treatment of choice is

a. Erythromycin
b. Supportive therapy
c. Trimethoprim-sulfamethoxazole
d. Cefuroxime

Items 8–10

A 19-year-old male presents with a 1-week history of malaise and anorexia followed by fever and sore throat. On physical examination, the throat is inflamed without exudate. There are a few palatal petechiae. Cervical adenopathy is present. The liver is percussed at 12 cm and the spleen is palpable.

Throat culture: negative for group A streptococci
Hct: 38%
Hgb: 12 g/dL
Reticulocytes: 4%
WBC: 14,000/μL
   Segmented: 30%
   Lymphocytes: 60%
   Monocytes: 10%
Bilirubin total: 2.0 mg/dL (normal 0.2 to 1.2)
Lactic dehydrogenase (LDH) serum: 260 IU/L (normal 20 to 220)
Aspartate (AST): 40 U/L (normal 8 to 20 U/L)
Alanine (ALT): 35 U/L (normal 8 to 20 U/L)
Alkaline phosphatase: 40 IU/L (normal 35 to 125)

8. The most important initial test is

a. Liver biopsy
b. Strep screen
c. Peripheral blood smear
d. Toxoplasmosis IgG
e. Lymph node biopsy

9. The most important serum test is

a. Heterophile antibody
b. Hepatitis B IgM
c. Cytomegalovirus IgG
d. ASLO titer
e. Hepatitis C antibody

10. Corticosteroids would be indicated if

a. Liver function tests worsen
b. Fatigue lasts more than 1 week
c. Severe hemolytic anemia is demonstrated
d. Hepatitis B is confirmed

DIRECTIONS: Each group of questions below consists of lettered options followed by a set of numbered items. For each numbered item, select the **one** lettered option with which it is **most** closely associated. Each lettered option may be used once, more than once, or not at all.

Items 11–14

Match the clinical description with the most likely organism.

a. *Streptococcus pneumoniae*
b. *Staphylococcus aureus*
c. Viridans streptococci
d. *Providencia stuartii*
e. *Actinomyces israelii*
f. *Haemophilus ducreyi*
g. *Neisseria meningitidis*
h. *Listeria monocytogenes*

11. A 30-year-old female with mitral valve prolapse and mitral regurgitant murmur develops fever, weight loss, and anorexia after undergoing a dental procedure. **(CHOOSE 1 ORGANISM)**

12. An 80-year-old-male, hospitalized for hip fracture, has a Foley catheter in place when he develops shaking chills, fever, and hypotension. **(CHOOSE 1 ORGANISM)**

13. A young man develops a painless, fluctuant purplish lesion over the mandible. Cutaneous fistula is noted after several weeks. **(CHOOSE 1 ORGANISM)**

14. A sickle cell anemia patient presents with high fever, toxicity, signs of pneumonia, and stiff neck. **(CHOOSE 1 ORGANISM)**

Items 15–18

Select an antiviral agent for each patient.
a. Ganciclovir
b. Acyclovir
c. Interferon α
d. Didanosine
e. Ribavirin
f. Amantadine
g. Vidarabine
h. Zalcitabine

15. A military recruit develops pneumonia secondary to influenza A. Symptoms began 24 h prior to physician visit. **(SELECT 1 AGENT)**

16. An HIV-positive patient with a CD4 count of 50 complains of the onset of visual blurring; opacity is seen on funduscopic exam. **(SELECT 1 AGENT)**

17. A sexually active young woman has anogenital warts and requests intralesional therapy. **(SELECT 1 AGENT)**

18. An infant with respiratory syncytial virus infection requires mechanical ventilation. **(SELECT 1 AGENT)**

Items 19–21

Select the fungal agent most likely responsible for the disease process described.
a. *Histoplasma capsulatum*
b. *Blastomycosis dermatitidis*
c. *Coccidioides immitis*
d. *Cryptococcus neoformans*
e. *Candida albicans*
f. *Aspergillus fumigatus*
g. *Zygomycosis*

19. A young, previously healthy male presents with verrucous skin lesions, bone pain, fever, cough, and weight loss. Chest x-ray shows nodular infiltrates. **(SELECT 1 AGENT)**

20. A diabetic patient is admitted with elevated blood sugar and acidosis. The patient complains of headache and sinus tenderness and has black, necrotic material draining from the nares. **(SELECT 1 AGENT)**

21. A young woman presents with asthma and eosinophilia. Fleeting pulmonary infiltrates occur with bronchial plugging. **(SELECT 1 AGENT)**

Items 22–24

A 40-year-old male develops bilateral facial weakness after returning from a camping trip in Wisconsin that lasted 6 weeks. The patient gives a history of arthralgias. On exam, he cannot close either eye well or raise either eyebrow. The first heart sound is diminished. There is no evidence of arthritis.

Hgb: 14 g/dL
WBC: 10,000/μL
VDRL: negative
FTA-Abs: positive
ECG: first-degree AV block

22. Which of the following would be most useful?

a. CT scan of head
b. MRI of head
c. More detailed history
d. Kveim test

23. The likely cause of these symptoms is

a. Intracranial infection
b. Lyme disease
c. Endocarditis
d. Herpes simplex

24. Treatment of choice is

a. Penicillin or ceftriaxone
b. Acyclovir
c. Corticosteroids
d. Aminoglycoside

25. You are a physician in charge of the patients who reside in a nursing home. Several of the patients have developed influenza-like symptoms, and the community is in the midst of an influenza A outbreak. None of the nursing home residents have received the influenza vaccine. What course of action is most appropriate?

a. Give the influenza vaccine to all residents who do not have a contraindication to the vaccine (i.e., allergy to eggs)
b. Give the influenza vaccine to all residents who do not have a contraindication to the vaccine; also give amantadine for 2 weeks
c. Give amantadine alone to all residents
d. Do not give any prophylactic regimen

26. An elderly male develops fever 3 days after cholecystectomy. He becomes short of breath, and chest x-ray shows a new right lower lobe infiltrate. Sputum Gram stain shows gram-positive cocci in clumps, and preliminary culture results suggest staphylococci. The initial antibiotic of choice is

a. Penicillinase-resistant penicillin such as nafcillin
b. Vancomycin
c. Antibiotic therapy should be based on the incidence of methicillin-resistant staphylococci in that hospital
d. Quinolones have become the drug of choice for pneumonia

27. A 30-year-old male with sickle cell anemia is admitted with cough, rusty sputum, and a single shaking chill. Physical examination reveals increased tactile fremitus and bronchial breath sounds in the left posterior chest. The patient is able to expectorate a purulent sample. Which of the following best describes the role of sputum Gram stain and culture?

a. Sputum Gram stain and culture lack the sensitivity and specificity to be of value in this setting
b. If the sample is a good one, sputum culture is useful in determining the antibiotic sensitivity pattern of the organism, particularly *Streptococcus pneumoniae*
c. Empirical use of antibiotics for pneumonia has made specific diagnosis unnecessary
d. There is no characteristic Gram stain in a patient with pneumococcal pneumonia

28. A 30-year-old man who has spent 5 of the last 10 years in prison in New York City is referred from the prison because of hemoptysis. He has a history of tuberculosis diagnosed 3 years ago and took isoniazid and rifampin for about a month. A cavitary lesion is seen on chest x-ray. The physician should do all the following except

a. Obtain sputum for acid-fast bacilli (AFB) stain, culture, and sensitivity
b. Start supervised isoniazid and rifampin administration
c. Start a supervised multiple drug combination to treat multidrug-resistant tuberculosis
d. Place the patient in respiratory isolation
e. Perform routine screening of inmates and staff for tuberculosis

29. A recent outbreak of severe diarrhea is currently being investigated. Several children developed bloody diarrhea, and one remains hospitalized with acute renal failure. A preliminary investigation has determined that all the affected children ate at the same restaurant. The food they consumed was most likely to be

a. Pork chops
b. Hamburger
c. Gefilte fish
d. Sushi
e. Soft-boiled eggs

30. A 40-year-old female nurse was admitted to the hospital because of fever to 103°F. Despite a thorough workup in the hospital for over 3 weeks, no etiology has been found, and she continues to have temperature spikes greater than 102°F. The least likely diagnosis in this patient is

a. Occult bacterial infection
b. Influenza
c. Lymphoma
d. Adult Still's disease
e. Factitious fever

31. In a patient who has mitral valve insufficiency, which procedure does not require prophylactic antibiotic therapy?

a. Cardiac catheterization
b. Prostatectomy
c. Cystoscopy
d. Tonsillectomy
e. Periodontal surgery

32. Rabies, an acute viral disease of the mammalian central nervous system, is transmitted by infective secretions, usually saliva. Which of the following statements about this disease is correct?

a. The disease is caused by a reovirus that elicits both complement-fixing and hemagglutinating antibodies useful in the diagnosis of the disease
b. The incubation period is variable, and, although 10 days is the most common elapsed time between infection and symptoms, some cases remain asymptomatic for 30 days
c. Only 30% of infected patients will survive
d. In the United States, the skunk and the raccoon have been important recent sources of human disease
e. Wild animals that have bitten and are suspected of being rabid should be killed and their brains examined for virus particles by electron microscopy

Items 33–36

Match each clinical description with the appropriate infectious agent.

a. Herpes simplex virus
b. Epstein-Barr virus
c. Parvovirus B19
d. *Staphylococcus aureus*
e. *Neisseria meningitidis*

33. Slapped-cheek rash

34. Desquamation of skin on hands and feet

35. Petechiae on trunk

36. Diffuse rash after administration of ampicillin

Items 37–41

Match the following diseases with their appropriate signs or associations.

a. Koplik spots
b. Agammaglobulinemia
c. A vesicular and pustular eruption that begins when the patient is afebrile
d. Acute cerebellar ataxia
e. Pancreatitis

37. Mumps **(CHOOSE 1 SIGN)**

38. Chickenpox **(CHOOSE 1 SIGN)**

39. Smallpox **(CHOOSE 1 SIGN)**

40. Echovirus infection **(CHOOSE 1 SIGN)**

41. Measles **(CHOOSE 1 SIGN)**

Items 42–46

Match the clinical illness with the appropriate opportunistic pathogen in patients with AIDS.

a. *Pneumocystis carinii*
b. *Toxoplasma gondii*
c. *Cryptosporidium*
d. Cytomegalovirus
e. *Salmonella*

42. Pneumonia **(CHOOSE 1 PATHOGEN)**

43. Retinitis **(CHOOSE 1 PATHOGEN)**

44. Seizures **(CHOOSE 1 PATHOGEN)**

45. Bacteremia **(CHOOSE 1 PATHOGEN)**

46. Diarrhea diagnosed by direct examination of stool **(CHOOSE 1 PATHOGEN)**

Items 47–51

For each of the sexually transmitted diseases, select the treatment of choice.

a. Penicillin
b. Doxycycline
c. Ceftriaxone plus doxycycline
d. Metronidazole
e. Acyclovir

47. Presumed gonococcal urethritis **(SELECT 1 TREATMENT)**

48. Nongonococcal urethritis **(SELECT 1 TREATMENT)**

49. Severe primary genital herpes **(SELECT 1 TREATMENT)**

50. Trichomoniasis **(SELECT 1 TREATMENT)**

51. Syphilis **(SELECT 1 TREATMENT)**

Items 52–55

Identify the antimicrobial agent associated with the adverse effects listed below.

a. Gentamicin
b. Imipenem
c. Tetracycline
d. Clindamycin

52. Photosensitivity **(CHOOSE 1 AGENT)**

53. Acute tubular necrosis **(CHOOSE 1 AGENT)**

54. Progressive weakness in a patient with myasthenia gravis **(CHOOSE 1 AGENT)**

55. Seizures **(CHOOSE 1 AGENT)**

56. A previously healthy 25-year-old music teacher develops fever and a rash over her face and chest. The rash is itchy and on exam involves multiple papules and vesicles in varying stages of development. One week later she complains of cough and is found to have an infiltrate on x-ray. The most likely etiology of the infection is

a. *Streptococcus pneumoniae*
b. *Mycoplasma pneumoniae*
c. *Pneumocystis carinii*
d. Varicella virus

Items 57–58

57. A 22-year-old male complains of fever and shortness of breath. There is no pleuritic chest pain or rigors and no sputum production. A chest x-ray shows diffuse perihilar infiltrates. The patient worsens while on erythromycin. A silver methenamine stain shows cystlike structures. Which of the following is correct?

a. Definitive diagnosis can be made by serology
b. The organism will grow after 48 h
c. History will likely provide important clues to the diagnosis
d. Cavitary disease is likely to develop

58. Which of the following statements about the treatment of the above patient is correct?

a. Oral antibiotic therapy is never appropriate
b. Trimethoprim-sulfamethoxazole is the treatment of choice in the nonallergic patient
c. Concomitant corticosteroids should always be avoided
d. Tetracycline is more effective than erythromycin

59. A 25-year-old male from East Tennessee had been ill for 5 days with fever, chills, and headache when he noted a rash that developed on his palms and soles. In addition to macular lesions, petechiae are noted on the wrists and ankles. The patient has spent the summer camping. The most important fact to be determined in the history is

a. Exposure to contaminated springwater
b. Exposure to raw pork
c. Exposure to ticks
d. Exposure to prostitutes

60. A 19-year-old male has a history of athlete's foot but is otherwise healthy when he develops the sudden onset of fever and pain in the right foot and leg. On physical exam, the foot and leg are fiery red with a well-defined indurated margin that appears to be rapidly advancing. There is tender inguinal lymphadenopathy. The most likely organism to cause this infection is

a. *Staphylococcus epidermidis*
b. *Tinea pedis*
c. *Streptococcus pyogenes*
d. Mixed anaerobic infection

61. An 18-year-old male has been seen in clinic for urethral discharge. He is treated with ceftriaxone, but the discharge has not resolved and the culture has returned as no growth. The most likely etiologic agent to cause this infection is

a. Ceftriaxone-resistant gonococci
b. *Chlamydia psittaci*
c. *Chlamydia trachomatis*
d. Herpes simplex

Items 62–68

Match the clinical description with the most likely etiologic agent.

a. *Candida albicans*
b. *Aspergillus flavus*
c. *Coccidioides immitis*
d. Herpes simplex type 1
e. Herpes simplex type 2
f. Hantavirus
g. *Tropheryma whippelii*
h. Coxsackievirus B
i. *Histoplasma capsulatum*
j. Human parvovirus
k. *Cryptococcus neoformans*

62. An HIV-positive patient develops fever and dysphagia; endoscopic biopsy shows yeast and hyphae. **(CHOOSE 1 AGENT)**

63. A 50-year-old develops sudden onset of bizarre behavior. CSF shows 80 lymphocytes; magnetic resonance imaging shows temporal lobe abnormalities. **(CHOOSE 1 AGENT)**

64. A patient with a previous history of tuberculosis now complains of hemoptysis. There is an upper lobe mass with a cavity and a crescent-shaped air-fluid level. **(CHOOSE 1 AGENT)**

65. A Filipino patient develops a pulmonary nodule after travel through the American Southwest. **(CHOOSE 1 AGENT)**

66. A 35-year-old male who had a fever, cough, and sore throat develops chest pain after several days with diffuse ST segment elevations on ECG. **(CHOOSE 1 AGENT)**

67. Overwhelming pneumonia with adult respiratory distress syndrome occurs on an Indian reservation in the Southwest following exposure to deer mice. **(CHOOSE 1 AGENT)**

68. A child develops an erythematous rash appearing as a slapped cheek. **(CHOOSE 1 AGENT)**

Infectious Disease

Answers

1. **The answer is c.** (*Gorbach, 2/e, pp 542–544.*) This patient, with the development of hoarseness, breathing difficulty, and stridor, is likely to have acute epiglottitis. Because of the possibility of impending airway obstruction, the patient should be admitted to an intensive care unit for close monitoring. The diagnosis can be confirmed by indirect laryngoscopy or soft tissue x-rays of the neck, which may show an enlarged epiglottis. Otolaryngology consult should be obtained. The most likely organism causing this infection is *Haemophilus influenzae*. Many of these organisms are β-lactamase-producing and would be resistant to ampicillin. The clinical findings are not consistent with the presentation of streptococcal pharyngitis. Lateral neck films would be more useful than a chest x-ray.

2. **The answer is a.** (*Braunwald, 15/e, p 190.*) Ear pain and drainage in an elderly diabetic patient must raise concern about malignant external otitis. The swelling and inflammation of the external auditory meatus strongly suggest this diagnosis. This infection usually occurs in older diabetics and is almost always caused by *P. aeruginosa*. *H. influenzae* and *M. catarrhalis* frequently cause otitis media, but not external otitis.

3–4. **The answers are 3-b, 4-a.** (*Braunwald, 15/e, pp 1046–1047.*) The diffuse rash involving palms and soles would in itself suggest the possibility of secondary syphilis. The hypertrophic, wartlike lesions around the anal area, called condylomata lata, are specific for secondary syphilis. The VDRL slide test will be positive in all patients with secondary syphilis. The Weil-Felix titer has been used as a screening test for rickettsial infection. In this patient, who has condylomata and no systemic symptoms, Rocky Mountain spotted fever would be unlikely. No chlamydial infection would present in this way. Blood cultures might be drawn to rule out bacterial infection such as chronic meningococcemia; however, the clinical picture is not consistent with a systemic bacterial infection. Penicillin is the drug of choice for secondary syphilis. Ceftriaxone and tetracycline are usually considered to be alternative therapies. Interferon α has been used in the treatment of condyloma acuminata, a lesion that can be mistaken for syphilitic condyloma.

5–7. The answers are 5-c, 6-b, 7-a. (*Braunwald, 15/e, pp 1073–1074.*) This young woman presents with symptoms of both upper and lower respiratory infection. The combination of sore throat, bullous myringitis, and infiltrates on chest x-ray is consistent with infection due to *M. pneumoniae*. This minute organism is not seen on Gram stain. Neither *S. pneumoniae* nor *H. influenzae* would produce this combination of upper and lower respiratory tract symptoms. The patient is likely to have high titers of IgM cold agglutinins. The low hematocrit and elevated reticulocyte count reflect a hemolytic anemia that can occur from mycoplasma infection. These IgM-class antibodies are directed to the I antigen on the erythrocyte membrane. The treatment of choice for mycoplasma infection is erythromycin.

8–10. The answers are 8-c, 9-a, 10-c. (*Braunwald, 15/e, pp 1109–1111.*) This young man presents with classic signs and symptoms of infectious mononucleosis. In a young patient with fever, pharyngitis, lymphadenopathy, and lymphocytosis, the peripheral blood smear should be evaluated for atypical lymphocytes. A heterophile antibody test should be performed. The symptoms described in association with atypical lymphocytes and a positive heterophile test are virtually always due to Epstein-Barr virus. Neither liver biopsy nor lymph node biopsy is necessary. Workup for toxoplasmosis or cytomegalovirus infection or hepatitis B and C would be considered in heterophile-negative patients, Hepatitis does not occur in the setting of rheumatic fever, and an antistreptolysin O titer is not indicated. Corticosteroids are indicated in the treatment of infectious mononucleosis when severe hemolytic anemia is demonstrated or when airway obstruction occurs. Neither fatigue nor the complication of hepatitis is an indication for corticosteroid therapy.

11–14. The answers are 11-c, 12-d, 13-e, 14-a. (*Braunwald, 15/e, pp 809–814, 882–885, 959, 1009, 1620.*) The 30-year-old-female with mitral valve prolapse has developed subacute bacterial endocarditis. The likely etiologic agent is a viridans streptococci. Viridans streptococci cause most cases of subacute bacterial endocarditis. No other agent listed is likely to cause this infection. The 80-year-old-male with a Foley catheter in place has developed a nosocomial infection likely secondary to urosepsis. *Providencia* species frequently cause urinary tract infection in the hospitalized patient. The young man with a fluctuant lesion and fistula over the mandible presents a classic picture of cervicofacial actinomycosis. The sickle cell anemia patient who presents with concomitant pneumonia and meningitis has overwhelming infection with S. pneumoniae due to functional asplenia. S. pneumoniae causes a particularly severe infection associated with sickle cell disease.

15–18. The answers are 15-f, 16-a, 17-c, 18-e. (Braunwald, 15/e, pp 1092–1100.) Amantadine has been shown to alter the course of influenza A favorably, particularly when begun within 48 h of the start of symptoms. The HIV-positive patient with a low CD4 count and visual blurring has developed cytomegalovirus retinitis. Gancyclovir is the drug of choice (foscarnet has also been used effectively). Interferon α has been approved for intralesional therapy of condyloma acuminatum (venereal warts caused by papillomavirus). Ribavirin improves mortality in mechanically ventilated infants with RSV infection.

19–21. The answers are 19-b, 20-g, 21-f. (Braunwald, 15/e, pp 1173–1179.) Blastomycosis presents with signs and symptoms of chronic respiratory infection. The organism has a tendency to produce skin lesions in exposed areas that become crusted, ulcerated, or verrucous. Bone pain is caused by osteolytic lesions. Mucormycosis is a zygomycosis that originates in the nose and paranasal sinuses. Sinus tenderness, bloody nasal discharge, and obtundation occur usually in the setting of diabetic ketoacidosis. *Aspergillus* can result in several different infectious processes, including aspergilloma, disseminated *Aspergillus* in the immunocompromised patient, or allergic bronchopulmonary aspergillosis. Bronchopulmonary aspergillosis is the most likely diagnosis in the young woman with asthma and eosinophilia. Bronchial plugs, often filled with hyphal forms, result in repeated infiltrates and exacerbation of wheezing.

22–24. The answers are 22-c, 23-b, 24-a. (Braunwald, 15/e, pp 1061–1065.) This patient presents with a symptom complex that includes facial nerve palsies, arthralgia, and first-degree AV block. Facial nerve palsy has been increasingly recognized as a first manifestation of Lyme disease. Within several weeks of the onset of illness, about 8% of patients develop cardiac involvement, with heart block being the most common manifestation. During this stage of early disseminated infection, musculoskeletal pain is common. The diagnosis of Lyme disease is based on careful history and physical exam with serologic confirmation by detection of antibody to

Borrelia burgdorferi. Neither CT or MRI of head would be indicated as the lesion is a peripheral facial palsy. Sarcoidosis can also cause both facial nerve palsy and AV block, but it is much less likely, and the Kveim test is rarely used to pursue this diagnosis. The treatment of choice for Lyme disease at this stage would be penicillin or ceftriaxone.

25. The answer is b. *(Braunwald, 15/e, pp 1125–1131.)* Influenza A is a potentially lethal disease in the elderly and chronically debilitated patient. In institutional settings such as nursing homes, outbreaks are likely to be particularly severe. Thus prophylaxis is extremely important in this setting. All residents should receive the vaccine unless they have known egg allergy (patients can choose to decline the vaccine). Since protective antibodies to the vaccine will not develop for 2 weeks, amantadine can be used for protection against influenza A during the interim 2-week period. A reduced dose is given to elderly patients.

26. The answer is c. *(Braunwald, 15/e, p 896.)* In the treatment of hospital-acquired staphylococcal pneumonia, the incidence of methicillin-resistant staph in the local facility will be very important. In most hospitals, methicillin-resistant staph is common enough to require initial therapy with vancomycin. Oxacillin would be the drug of choice only if the incidence of methicillin-resistant staph is very low. Quinolones are often useful in the treatment of community-acquired pneumonia, but they would not be effective against methicillin-resistant staph.

27. The answer is b. *(Braunwald, 15/e, p 1479.)* The Infectious Disease Society of America's guidelines on the treatment of community-acquired pneumonia still recommend the use of sputum gram stain and culture. This is particularly important in the era of multi-antibiotic-resistant *S. pneumoniae.* Sputum culture and sensitivity can direct specific antibiotic therapy for the patient as well as provide epidemiologic information for the community as a whole. A good sputum sample showing many polymorphonuclear leukocytes and few squamous epithelial cells can give important clues to etiology. A Gram stain that shows gram-positive lancet-shaped diplococci intracellularly is good evidence for pneumococcal infection. Empirical antibiotic therapy becomes more difficult in community-acquired pneumonia as more pathogens are recognized and as the pneumococcus develops resistance to penicillin, macrolides, and even quinolones.

28. The answer is b. (*Braunwald, 15/e, pp 1031–1034.*) Multidrug-resistant tuberculosis (TB) has become an increasing problem in several settings, including correctional facilities and health care institutions. Noncompliance or poor compliance with prescribed anti-TB medications is the major factor in the development of multiple drug resistance. When the disease is suspected, patients should be placed in respiratory isolation and sputum should be obtained for AFB stain, culture, and sensitivity. Treatment of high-risk patients, such as this patient, should be supervised, and multidrug resistance should be assumed. Regular screening of inmates and staff for TB is important for preventing the spread of TB within the facility and for early diagnosis of new infections.

29. The answer is b. (*Braunwald, 15/e, pp 242, 954.*) The outbreak described is similar to those previously attributed to *Escherichia coli* 0157:H7. Ingestion of and infection with this organism may result in a spectrum of illnesses, including mild diarrhea, hemorrhagic colitis with bloody diarrhea, acute renal failure, and death. Infection has been associated with ingestion of contaminated beef (in particular ground beef), ingestion of raw milk, and contamination via the fecal-oral route. Cooking ground beef so that it is no longer pink is an effective means of preventing infection, as are hand washing and pasteurization of milk.

30. The answer is b. (*Stobo, 23/e, pp 547–551.*) Patients may develop fever as a result of infectious or noninfectious diseases. The term *fever of unknown origin* (FUO) is applied when significant fever persists without a known cause after an adequate evaluation. Several studies have found the leading causes of FUO to include infections, malignancies, collagen vascular diseases, and granulomatous diseases. As the ability to more rapidly diagnose some of these diseases increases, their likelihood of causing undiagnosed persistent fever lessens. Infections such as intraabdominal abscesses, tuberculosis, hepatobiliary disease, endocarditis (especially if the patient had previously taken antibiotics), and osteomyelitis may cause FUO. In immunocompromised patients, such as those infected with HIV, a number of opportunistic infections or lymphomas may cause fever and escape early diagnosis. Self-limited infections such as influenza should not cause fever that persists for many weeks. Neoplastic diseases such as lymphomas and some solid tumors (e.g., hypernephroma and primary or metastatic disease of the liver) are associated with FUO. A number of collagen vascular diseases may cause FUO. Since conditions such as systemic lupus erythematosus are more easily diagnosed today, they are less frequent causes of this syndrome. Adult Still's disease, however, is often difficult to diagnose. Other causes of FUO include granulomatous diseases (i.e., giant cell arteritis, regional enteritis, sarcoidosis, and granulomatous hepatitis), drug fever, and peripheral pulmonary emboli. Factitious fever is most common among young adults employed in health-related positions. A prior psychiatric history or multiple hospitalizations at other institutions may be clues to this condition. Such patients may induce infections by self-injection of nonsterile material, with resultant multiple abscesses or polymicrobial infections. Alternatively, some patients may manipulate their thermometers. In these cases, a discrepancy between temperature and pulse or between oral temperature and witnessed rectal temperature will be observed.

31. The answer is a. (*Mandell, 5/e, pp 917–923.*) Although no evidence exists that prophylactic antibiotic therapy prevents endocarditis, prophylaxis is recommended for all procedures that may generate bacteremias. Following cardiac catheterization, blood cultures obtained from a distal vein are rarely positive. Thus, prophylactic antibiotics are not currently recommended for cardiac catheterization. Bacteremia commonly occurs following other procedures such as periodontal surgery, tonsillectomy, and prostate surgery.

32. The answer is d. (*Mandell, 5/e, pp 1811–1819.*) Rabies is caused by a bullet-shaped rhabdovirus. In the United States, dogs are seldom rabid. The animals that present the most danger are wild skunks and bats; foxes are also possible carriers. Raccoons are responsible for an increasing number of cases in the mid-Atlantic states. The incubation period ranges from 4 days to many years, but is usually between 20 and 90 days. The incubation period is usually shorter with a bite to the head than with one to an extremity. In humans, only four definite recoveries from established infection have been reported. Nonimmunized animals that have been bitten should be killed and their brains submitted for virus by immunofluorescent antibody examination. A negative fluorescent test removes the need to treat the bite victim either actively or passively.

33–36. The answers are 33-c, 34-d, 35-e, 36-b. (*Gorbach, 2/e, pp 1334–1335, 1387, 1648, 1692.*) Parvovirus B19 is the agent responsible for erythema infectiosum, also known as fifth disease. This disease most commonly affects children between the ages of 5 and 14 years, but it can also occur in adults. The disease is characterized by a slapped-cheek rash, which may follow a prodrome of low-grade fever. A diffuse lacelike rash may also occur. Complications in adults include arthralgias, arthritis, aplastic crisis in patients with chronic hemolytic anemia, spontaneous abortion, and hydrops fetalis. Desquamation of the skin usually occurs during or after recovery from toxic shock syndrome (associated with a toxin produced by *S. aureus*). Peeling of the skin is also seen in Kawasaki disease, scarlet fever, and some severe drug reactions. Petechial rashes are often seen with potentially life-threatening infections, including meningococcemia, gonococcemia, rickettsial disease, infective endocarditis, atypical measles, and disseminated intravascular coagulation (DIC) associated with sepsis. Infectious mononucleosis is the usual manifestation of infection with Epstein-Barr virus. Since it is a viral disease, antibiotic therapy is not indicated. A diffuse maculopapular rash has been observed in over 90% of patients with infectious mononucleosis who are given ampicillin. The rash does not represent an allergic reaction to β-lactam antibiotics.

37–41. The answers are 37-e, 38-d, 39-c, 40-b, 41-a. (*Mandell, 5/e, pp 1555, 1776–1780, 1801–1807.*) Although salivary adenitis is the most prominent feature of the communicable disease of viral origin, mumps, involvement of the gonads, meninges, and pancreas is not uncommon. Males who develop mumps after puberty have a 20 to 35% chance of developing a painful orchitis. Central nervous system involvement is common but usually mild, with 50% of cases causing an increase in lymphocytes detectable in the CSF. Myocarditis, thrombocytopenic purpura, and polyarthritis may also occur as complications of this disease. An inflammatory change in the pancreas is a potentially serious problem; symptoms consist of abdominal discomfort and a gastroenteritis-like illness. Although a polyneuritis and a transverse myelitis have been described, the most common manifestation of CNS infection with varicella (chickenpox) is acute cerebellar ataxia. While chickenpox is usually a benign illness in children, other complications such as myocarditis, iritis, nephritis, orchitis, and hepatitis may occur. Pneumonitis occurs more commonly in adults than children.

It can be difficult to distinguish between the vesicular lesions of small-pox and chickenpox. Classically, however, a history of rash with vesicles that develop over a few hours would be typical of a chickenpox infection; vesiculation that develops over a period of days is the rule in smallpox. While fever is characteristic of the prodrome of smallpox, it subsides prior to focal eruptions. Lesions of smallpox are typically all at the same stage of development, in contrast to the various stages seen in a patient with chickenpox. Preparations of vesicular fluid under electron microscopy show characteristic brick-shaped particles with poxvirus. A more readily available test, the Tzanck smear, performed by scraping the base of the lesion, should reveal multinucleated giant cells microscopically in a patient with chickenpox. Humoral immunity appears to be very important in the recovery from enteroviral infections. One of the most common complications for patients with sex-linked or acquired agammaglobulinemia is a chronic central nervous system infection with an echovirus. In the absence of the ability to produce antibodies, this virus spreads rapidly and usually produces a fatal illness. The administration of intravenous preparations of gamma globulin intraventricularly has controlled this serious complication of immune deficiency in some patients.

It may take from 9 to 11 days after exposure for the first symptoms of measles to develop. Malaise, irritability, and a high fever often associated with conjunctivitis with prominent tearing are common symptoms. This prodromal syndrome may last from 3 days to 1 week before the characteristic rash of measles develops. One or two days before the onset of the rash, characteristic Koplik spots (small, red, irregular lesions with blue-white centers) may be visible on the mucous membranes and occasionally on the conjunctiva. Classically, the measles rash will begin on the forehead and spread downward, and the Koplik spots will rapidly resolve.

42–46. The answers are 42-a, 43-d, 44-b, 45-e, 46-c. *(Braunwald, 15/e, pp 1880–1896.)* Pneumonia due to *P. carinii* was among the first recognized manifestations of AIDS. The chest radiograph typically shows a diffuse bilateral interstitial pattern, but other patterns, including a normal radiograph, may occur. *Pneumocystis* infection may also occur at extrapulmonary sites. Cytomegalovirus (CMV) is a frequent disseminated pathogen that causes retinitis that may lead to blindness. CMV may also cause pneumonitis, adrenalitis, and hepatitis, as well as colitis with significant diarrhea. The protozoan *Cryptosporidium* may cause a chronic diarrhea that leads to malabsorption and wasting. It can be diagnosed by direct examination of the stool with special concentration or staining techniques or both. *Salmonella* infections have been recognized with increased frequency in patients with HIV. These patients are typically bacteremic and develop bacteremic relapse; they do not usually present with a diarrheal illness. Patients who present with seizures warrant evaluation for toxoplasmosis. CNS lymphoma and certain other infections may also cause seizures. Patients with toxoplasmic encephalitis may also have toxoplasmic chorioretinitis, although CMV remains the most common identified cause of retinitis in patients with AIDS.

47–51. The answers are 47-c, 48-b, 49-e, 50-d, 51-a. (*Braunwald, 15/e, pp 936–937, 1050–1052, 1230.*) Treatment of gonococcal infections should be guided by the increasing frequency of antibiotic-resistant *Neisseria gonorrhoeae* and high frequency of co-infection with *Chlamydia trachomatis*. Because of the increased frequency of resistance to penicillin and tetracyclines, ceftriaxone is recommended as the treatment of choice. Doxycycline is added to treat chlamydial and other causes of nongonococcal urethritis. First episodes of genital herpes may be particularly severe. Oral acyclovir will accelerate the healing but will not reduce the risk of recurrence once the drug is stopped. Trichomoniasis is usually diagnosed by a wet preparation microscopic examination or by culture. Both the patient and sexual partner should be treated with metronidazole. Penicillin remains the drug of choice for treatment of syphilis. The route of administration and duration of therapy depend on the stage of disease and presence of CNS involvement and may also be influenced by the HIV serostatus of the patient.

52–55. The answers are 52-c, 53-a, 54-a, 55-b. (*Braunwald, 15/e, pp 875–882.*) The tetracyclines are associated with photosensitization, and patients taking these antibiotics should be warned about exposure to the sun. Imipenem, a carbapenem, may cause central nervous system toxicity such as seizures, especially when administered at high dosages. The major toxicity of gentamicin, an aminoglycoside, is acute tubular necrosis; thus, drug levels should be closely monitored. The aminoglycosides may be ototoxic, with effects on vestibular or auditory function or both. This class of drugs can also produce neuromuscular blockade, especially when administered with concomitant neuromuscular blocking agents or to patients with impairment of neuromuscular transmission, such as myasthenia gravis.

56. The answer is d. *(Braunwald, 15/e, p 1107.)* Varicella pneumonia develops in about 20% of adults with chickenpox. It occurs 3 to 7 days after the onset of the rash. The hallmark of the chickenpox rash is papules, vesicles, and scabs in various stages of development. Fever, malaise, and itching are usually part of the clinical picture. The differential can include some coxsackievirus and echovirus infections, which might present with pneumonia and vesicular rash. Rickettsialpox, a rickettsial infection, has also been mistaken for chickenpox.

57. The answer is c. *(Braunwald, 15/e, pp 1182–1184.)* Patients with *P. carinii* pneumonia frequently present with shortness of breath and no sputum production. The interstitial pattern of infiltrates on chest x-ray distinguishes the pneumonia from most bacterial infections. Diagnosis is made by review of silver methenamine stain. Serology is not sensitive or specific enough for routine use. The organism does not grow on any media. Cavitation can occur but is quite unusual. The history is likely to suggest a risk factor for HIV disease.

58. The answer is b. *(Gantz, 4/e, pp 455–459.)* Trimethoprim-sulfa is the drug of choice for *P. carinii* pneumonia in the nonallergic patient. Oral therapy is recommended for mild to moderate disease. Prednisone has been shown to improve the mortality rate in moderate to severe disease when the PO_2 is less than 70 mmHg. Neither tetracycline nor erythromycin has any effect on the organism.

59. The answer is c. *(Braunwald, 15/e, pp 1065–1066.)* The rash of Rocky Mountain spotted fever (RMSF) occurs about 5 days into an illness characterized by fever, malaise, and headache. The rash may be macular or petechial, but almost always spreads from the ankles and wrists to the trunk. The disease is most common in spring and summer. North Carolina and East Tennessee have a relatively high index of disease. RMSF is a rickettsial disease with the tick as the vector. About 80% of patients will give a history of tick exposure. Doxycycline is considered the drug of choice, but chloramphenicol is preferred in pregnancy because of the effects of tetracycline on fetal bones and teeth. Overall mortality from the infection is now about 5%.

60. The answer is c. (*Braunwald, 15/e, pp 823, 893.*) Erysipelas, the cellulitis described, is typical of infection caused by *S. pyogenes* group A β-hemolytic streptococci. There is often a preceding event such as a cut in the skin, dermatitis, or superficial fungal infection that precedes this rapidly spreading cellulitis. Anaerobic cellulitis is more often associated with underlying diabetes. *S. epidermidis* does not cause rapidly progressive cellulitis. *Staphylococcus aureus* can cause cellulitis that is difficult to distinguish from erysipelas, but it is usually more focal and likely to produce furuncles, or abscesses.

61. The answer is c. (*Braunwald, 15/e, pp 1074–1076, 1620–1622.*) About half of all cases of nongonococcal urethritis are caused by *C. trachomatis*. *Ureaplasma urealyticum* and *Trichomonas vaginalis* are rarer causes of urethritis. Herpes simplex would present with vesicular lesions and pain. *C. psittaci* is the etiologic agent in psittacosis. All gonococci are susceptible to ceftriaxone at recommended doses.

62–68. The answers are 62-a, 63-d, 64-b, 65-c, 66-h, 67-f, 68-j. (*Gorbach, 2/e, pp 592, 1334–1335, 2094–2095, 2142, 2164–2168, 2314–2315, 2327–2329.*) There are several causes for dysphagia in the HIV-positive patient, including *C. albicans*, herpes simplex, and cytomegalovirus. The biopsy result in this patient confirms *Candida* infection with the typical picture of both yeast and hyphae seen on smear. Herpes simplex encephalitis can occur in patients of any age—usually in immunocompetent patients. The bizarre behavior includes personality aberrations, hypersexuality, or sensory hallucinations. CSF shows lymphocytes with a close to normal sugar and protein. Focal abnormalities are seen in the temporal lobe by CT scan, MRI, or EEG.

The patient who has had a previous history of tuberculosis and now complains of hemoptysis would be reevaluated for active tuberculosis. However, the chest x-ray described is characteristic of a fungus ball—almost always the result of an aspergilloma.

The Filipino patient who has developed a pulmonary nodule after travel through the Southwest would be suspected of having developed coccidioidomycosis. Individuals from the Philippines have a higher incidence of the disease and are more likely to have complications of dissemination.

The 35-year-old with cough, sore throat, and fever went on to develop symptoms of myopericarditis with typical ECG findings. Coxsackievirus B infection is the most likely cause of URI symptoms that evolve into a picture of myocarditis. Myocarditis may be asymptomatic or can present with chest pain, both pleuritic and ischemic-like. Enteroviruses rarely if ever attack the pericardium alone without involving the subepicardial myocardium.

Hantavirus pulmonary syndrome begins with a prodromal illness of cough, fever, and myalgias that is difficult to distinguish from other viral illnesses such as influenza. However, the illness progresses to increased dyspnea, hypoxia, and hypotension. The picture resembles adult respiratory distress syndrome (ARDS), and most patients require mechanical ventilation. The infection should be suspected when a previously healthy adult develops unexplained pulmonary edema or ARDS without known causes. Thrombocytopenia is also a useful clue. Transmission of hantavirus usually occurs through acrosolization of urine from infected rodents or through the bite of an infected rodent.

The slapped-cheek appearance in the child, previously called fifth disease, is now known to be the result of a parvovirus B19. Its occurrence may be epidemic in nature. Children are usually not very ill, but adults can develop a polyarthralgia or true arthritis.

Rheumatology

Questions

DIRECTIONS: Each item below contains a question or incomplete statement followed by suggested responses. Select the **one best** response to each question.

Items 69–70

69. A 40-year-old female complains of 7 weeks of pain and swelling in both wrists and knees. The patient complained of fatigue and lethargy several weeks before noticing the joint pain. The patient notes that after a period of rest, resistance to movement is more striking. On exam, the metacarpophalangeal joints and wrists are warm and tender. There are no other joint abnormalities. There is no alopecia, photosensitivity, kidney disease, or rash. Which of the following is correct?

a. The clinical picture suggests early rheumatoid arthritis, and a rheumatoid factor should be obtained
b. The prodrome of lethargy suggests chronic fatigue syndrome
c. Lack of systemic symptoms suggests osteoarthritis
d. X-rays of the hand are likely to show joint space narrowing and erosion

70. On follow-up, the patient continues to complain of joint stiffness over several months. In addition to swelling of the wrists and MCPs, tenderness and joint effusion has occurred in both knees. The rheumatoid factor has become positive, and subcutaneous nodules are noted on the extensor surfaces of the forearm. Which of the following statements is correct?

a. Corticosteroids should be started
b. The patient meets the American College of Rheumatology criteria for RA and should be evaluated for disease-modifying antirheumatic therapy
c. A nonsteroidal anti-inflammatory drug should be added to aspirin
d. The patient's prognosis is highly favorable

71. A 60-year-old female complains of dry mouth and a gritty sensation in her eyes. She states it is sometimes difficult to speak for more than a few minutes. There is no history of diabetes mellitus or neurologic disease. The patient is on no medications. On exam, the buccal mucosa appears dry and the salivary glands are enlarged bilaterally. The next step in evaluation is

a. Lip biopsy
b. Schirmer test and measurement of autoantibodies
c. IgG antibody to mumps virus
d. Use of corticosteroids

72. A 40-year-old male complains of exquisite pain and tenderness over the left ankle. There is no history of trauma. The patient is taking a mild diuretic for hypertension. On exam, the ankle is very swollen and tender. There are no other physical exam abnormalities. The next step in management is

a. Begin colchicine and broad-spectrum antibiotics
b. Obtain uric acid level and perform arthrocentesis
c. Begin allopurinol if uric acid level is elevated
d. Obtain ankle x-ray to rule out fracture

Items 73–74

73. A 70-year-old, non–sexually active male complains of fever and pain in his left knee. Several days previously, the patient skinned his knee while working in his garage. The knee is red, warm, and swollen. An arthocentesis is performed, which shows 200,000 leukocytes/μL and a glucose of 20 mg/dL. No crystals are noted. The most important next step is

a. Gram stain and culture of joint fluid
b. Urethral culture
c. Uric acid level
d. Antinuclear antibody

74. The most likely organism to cause septic arthritis in the case above is

a. *Streptococcus pneumoniae*
b. *Neisseria gonorrhoeae*
c. *Escherichia coli*
d. *Staphylococcus aureus*

75. A 50-year-old male complains of low back pain and stiffness, which becomes worse on bending and is relieved by lying down. There are no symptoms of fever, chills, weight loss, or urinary problems. He has had similar pain several years ago. On exam, there is paraspinal tenderness and spasm of the lower lumbar back. There are no sensory deficits, and reflexes are normal. The next step in management is

a. Lumbosacral spine films
b. Stretching exercises
c. Weight training
d. Activity as tolerated, optional 2-day bedrest
e. MRI

76. A 60-year-old male complains of pain in both knees coming on gradually over the past 2 years. The pain is relieved by rest and worsened by the movement. There is bony enlargement of the knees with mild inflammation. Crepitation is noted on motion of the knee joint. There are no other findings except for bony enlargement at the distal interphalangeal joint. The patient is 5 feet 9 in. tall and weighs 190 lb. The best way to prevent disease progression is

a. Weight reduction
b. Calcium supplementation
c. Total knee replacement
d. Aspirin
e. Oral prednisone

77. A 22-year-old male develops the insidious onset of low back pain improved with exercise and worsened by rest. There is no history of diarrhea, conjunctivitis, urethritis, eye problems, or nail changes. On exam the patient has loss of mobility with respect to lumbar flexion and extension. He has a kyphotic posture. A plain film of the spine shows widening and sclerosis of the sacroiliac joints. Some calcification is noted in the anterior spinal ligament. Which of the following best characterizes this patient's disease process?

a. He is most likely to have acute lumbosacral back strain and requires bed rest
b. The patient has a spondyloarthropathy, most likely ankylosing spondylitis
c. The patient is likely to die from pulmonary fibrosis and extrathoracic restrictive lung disease
d. A rheumatoid factor is likely to be positive
e. A colonoscopy is likely to show Crohn's disease

78. A 20-year-old woman has developed low-grade fever, a malar rash, and arthralgias of the hands over several months. High titers of anti-DNA antibodies are noted, and complement levels are low. The patient's white blood cell count is 3000/µL, and platelet count is 90,000/µL. The patient is on no medications and has no signs of active infection. Which of the following statements is correct?

a. If glomerulonephritis, severe thrombocytopenia, or hemolytic anemia develops, high-dose glucocorticoid therapy would be indicated
b. Central nervous system symptoms will occur within 10 years
c. The patient can be expected to develop Raynaud's phenomenon when exposed to cold
d. The patient will have a false-positive test for syphilis
e. The disease process described is an absolute contraindication to pregnancy

79. A 45-year-old woman has pain in her fingers on exposure to cold, arthralgias, and difficulty swallowing solid food. The most useful test to make a definitive diagnosis is

a. Rheumatoid factor
b. Antinucleolar antibody
c. ECG
d. BUN and creatinine

80. A 20-year-old male complains of arthritis and eye irritation. He has a history of burning on urination. On exam, there is a joint effusion of the right knee and a dermatitis of the glans penis. Which of the following is correct?

a. *Neisseria gonorrhoeae* is likely to be cultured from the glans penis
b. The patient is likely to be rheumatoid factor positive
c. An infectious process of the GI tract may precipitate this disease
d. An ANA is very likely to be positive

Items 81–82

81. A 75-year-old male complains of unilateral headache. On one occasion he transiently lost his vision. He also complains of aching in the shoulders and neck. There are no focal neurologic findings. Carotid pulses are normal without bruit. There is some tenderness over the left temple. Laboratory data show a mild anemia. Which of the following tests is most likely to be abnormal?

a. Carotid ultrasound
b. CT scan
c. Erythrocyte sedimentation rate
d. X-ray of the left shoulder
e. Skull films

82. In the above patient, who is shown to have an elevated ESR, the best approach to management is

a. Begin glucocorticoid therapy and arrange for temporal artery biopsy
b. Schedule biopsy and begin corticosteroids based on biopsy results and clinical course
c. Schedule carotid angiography
d. Follow ESR and consider further studies if it remains elevated

Items 83–84

83. A 65-year-old male develops the sudden onset of severe knee pain. The knee is red, swollen, and tender. He has a history of diabetes mellitus and cardiomyopathy. An x-ray of the knee shows linear calcification. Definitive diagnosis is best made by

a. Serum uric acid
b. Serum calcium
c. Arthrocentesis and identification of positively birefringent rhomboid crystals
d. Rheumatoid factor

84. Further workup in this patient should include evaluation for

a. Renal disease
b. Hemochromatosis
c. Peptic ulcer disease
d. Lyme disease

85. A 35-year-old woman complains of aching all over. She says she sleeps poorly and all her joints hurt. Symptoms have progressed over several years. Physical exam shows multiple points of tenderness over the neck, shoulders, elbows, and wrists. There is no joint swelling or deformity. A complete blood count and erythrocyte sedimentation rate are normal. Rheumatoid factor is negative. There is no tenderness over the median third of the clavicle, the medial malleolus, or the forehead. The best therapeutic option in this patient is

a. Amitriptyline at night
b. Prednisone
c. Aspirin and methotrexate
d. Plaquenil

86. A 70-year-old female with mild dementia complains of hip pain. There is some limitation of motion in the right hip. The first step in evaluation is

a. CBC and erythrocyte sedimentation rate
b. Rheumatoid factor
c. X-ray of right hip
d. Bone scan

DIRECTIONS: Each group of questions below consists of lettered options followed by a set of numbered items. For each numbered item select the **one** lettered option with which it is **most** closely associated. Each lettered option may be used once, more than once, or not at all.

Items 87–90

Select the most probable diagnosis for each patient.

a. Behçet syndrome
b. Ankylosing spondylitis
c. Polymyalgia rheumatica
d. Reiter syndrome
e. Drug-induced lupus erythematosus
f. Polyarteritis nodosa
g. Scleroderma

87. A 50-year-old drug abuser presents with fever and weight loss. Exam shows hypertension, nodular skin rash, and peripheral neuropathy. ESR is 100 mm/L, and RBC casts are seen on urinalysis. **(SELECT 1 DIAGNOSIS)**

88. An elderly male presents with pain in his shoulders and hands. ESR is 105 mm/L. History includes transient blindness and unilateral headache. **(SELECT 1 DIAGNOSIS)**

89. A young male presents with leg swelling and recurrent aphthous ulcers of his lips and tongue. He has also recently noted painful genital ulcers. There is no urethritis or conjunctivitis. On exam, he has evidence of deep vein thrombophlebitis. **(SELECT 1 DIAGNOSIS)**

90. A 19-year-old male complains of low back morning stiffness, pain, and limitation of motion of shoulders. He has eye pain and photophobia. Diastolic murmur is present on physical exam. **(SELECT 1 DIAGNOSIS)**

91. A 65-year-old woman who has a 12-year history of symmetrical polyarthritis is admitted to the hospital. Physical examination reveals splenomegaly, ulcerations over the lateral malleoli, and synovitis of the wrists, shoulders, and knees. There is no hepatomegaly. Laboratory values demonstrate a white blood cell count of 2500/µL and a rheumatoid factor titer of 1:4096. This patient's white blood cell differential count is likely to reveal

a. Pancytopenia
b. Lymphopenia
c. Granulocytopenia
d. Lymphocytosis
e. Basophilia

Items 92–96

For each side effect, select the drug with which it is closely associated.

a. Acetylsalicylic acid (aspirin)
b. Gold
c. Prednisone
d. Chloroquine
e. None of the above

92. Gastrointestinal bleeding **(SELECT 1 DRUG)**

93. Osteoporosis **(SELECT 1 DRUG)**

94. Retinopathy **(SELECT 1 DRUG)**

95. Proteinuria **(SELECT 1 DRUG)**

96. Stomatitis **(SELECT 1 DRUG)**

Items 97–101

Match each description with the appropriate disease.

a. Polyarteritis nodosa
b. Wegener's granulomatosis
c. Giant cell arteritis
d. Multiple cholesterol embolization syndrome
e. Takayasu's arteritis

97. Involvement of the upper and lower respiratory tracts; a cause of glomerulonephritis **(CHOOSE 1 DISEASE)**

98. Ecchymoses and necrosis in extremities in elderly patients **(CHOOSE 1 DISEASE)**

99. Inflammation of small- to medium-sized muscular arteries, which may cause kidney, heart, liver, gastrointestinal, and muscular damage **(CHOOSE 1 DISEASE)**

100. Occurs in patients above the age of 55, who may experience fever, weight loss, scalp pain, headache, and visual changes **(CHOOSE 1 DISEASE)**

101. Inflammation of the aorta and its branches in young women; also known as pulseless disease **(CHOOSE 1 DISEASE)**

102. A 50-year-old white female presents with aching and stiffness in the trunk, hip, and shoulders. There is widespread muscle pain after mild exertion. Symptoms are worse in the morning and improve during the day. They are also worsened by stress. The patient is always tired and exhausted. She has trouble sleeping at night. On exam, joints are normal but there are multiple points of tenderness over the occiput, neck, lateral epicondyle, and medial fat pad of the knee. ESR is normal, and there is no history of Lyme disease or HIV disease exposure. A definitive diagnosis is best made by

a. Trial of glucocorticoids
b. Muscle biopsy
c. Demonstration of 11 tender points
d. Psychiatric evaluation

103. A 35-year-old construction worker presents with complaints of nocturnal parasthesias of the thumb and the index and middle fingers. There is some atrophy of the thenar eminence. Tinel sign is positive. The most likely diagnosis is

a. Carpal tunnel syndrome
b. De Quervain's tenosynovitis
c. Amyotrophic lateral sclerosis
d. Rheumatoid arthritis of the wrist joint

Rheumatology

Answers

69. The answer is a. *(Braunwald, 15/e, pp 1933–1934.)* The clinical picture of symmetrical swelling and tenderness of the metacarpophalangeal (MCP) and wrist joints lasting longer than 6 weeks strongly suggests rheumatoid arthritis. Rheumatoid factor, an immunoglobulin directed against the Fc portion of IgG, is positive in about two-thirds of cases and is present early in the disease. The history of lethargy or fatigue is a common prodrome of RA. The inflammatory joint changes are not consistent with chronic fatigue syndrome. The MCP-wrist distribution of joint symptoms makes osteoarthritis very unlikely. The x-ray changes described are characteristic of RA, but would occur later in the course of the disease.

70. The answer is b. *(Braunwald, 15/e, pp 1934–1936.)* The patient has more than four of the required signs or symptoms of RA, including morning stiffness, swelling of the wrist or MCP, simultaneous swelling of joints on both sides of body, subcutaneous nodules, and positive rheumatoid factor. Subcutaneous nodules are a poor prognostic sign for the activity of the disease, and disease-modifying drugs (gold, penicillamine, antimalarials, or methotrexate) should be instituted. Methotrexate has emerged as the agent of choice. Oral corticosteroids are generally withheld unless absolutely necessary and after disease-modifying drugs are instituted. However, low-dose corticosteroids have recently been shown to reduce the progression of bony erosions. There is no value to using both aspirin and nonsteroidals together, as simultaneous usage will increase side effects.

71. The answer is b. *(Braunwald, 15/e, pp 1947–1949.)* The complaints described are characteristic of Sjögren syndrome, an autoimmune disease with presenting symptoms of dry eyes and dry mouth. The disease is caused by lymphocytic infiltration and destruction of lacrimal and salivary glands. Dry eyes can be measured objectively by the Schirmer test, which measures the amount of wetness of a piece of filter paper when exposed to the lower eyelid for 5 minutes. Most patients with Sjögren syndrome produce autoantibodies, particularly anti-Ro (SSA). Lip biopsy is needed only to evaluate uncertain cases, such as when dry mouth occurs without dry eye symptoms. Mumps can cause bilateral parotitis, but would not explain the patient's dry eye syndrome. Corticosteroids are reserved for life-threatening vasculitis, particularly when renal or pulmonary disease is severe.

72. The answer is b. (*Braunwald, 15/e, pp 1994–1995.*) The sudden onset and severity of this monoarticular arthritis suggests acute gouty arthritis, especially in a patient on diuretic therapy. However, an arthrocentesis is indicated in the first episode to document gout by demonstrating needle-shaped, negatively birefringent crystals and to rule out other diagnoses such as infection. For most patients with acute gout, NSAIDs are the treatment of choice. Colchicine is also effective, but causes nausea and diarrhea. Antibiotics should not be started for infectious arthritis before an arthrocentesis is performed. Hyperuricemia should never be treated in the setting of an acute attack of gouty arthritis. Long-term goals of management are to control hyperuricemia, prevent further attacks, and prevent joint damage. Long-term prophylaxis with a uricosuric agent or allopurinol is considered for repeated attacks of acute arthritis, urolithiasis, or formation of tophaceous deposits. Attempts to normalize serum uric acid prior to drug therapy should include control of body weight, avoidance of ethanol and diuretics, and perhaps low-purine diet. X-ray of the ankle would likely be inconclusive in this patient with no trauma history.

73. The answer is a. (*Stobo, 23/e, pp 251–256.*) The clinical and laboratory picture suggests an acute septic arthritis. The most important first step is to determine the etiologic agent of the infection. Gout would be unlikely to produce the 200,000 leukocytes in the joint fluid. There is no history of symptoms suggesting connective tissue disease. Gonococci can cause a septic arthritis, but a urethral culture in the absence of urethral discharge would not be helpful.

74. The answer is d. (*Braunwald, 15/e, pp 895, 1998.*) *S. aureus* is the most common organism to cause septic arthritis in adults. β-hemolytic streptococci are the second most common. *N. gonorrhoeae* can also produce septic arthritis, but would be less likely in this patient who is not sexually active. *S. pneumoniae* and *E. coli* are rare causes of septic arthritis and usually occur secondary to a primary focus of infection.

75. The answer is d. *(Braunwald, 15/e, pp 85–87.)* The patient presents with symptoms consistent with acute mechanical low back pain. Even patients with lumbar disc herniation and sciatica improve with nonoperative care, and imaging studies do not affect initial management. Activity as tolerated with optional 2 days of bed rest is recommended along with adequate pain control and reassurance. Active therapy to restore range of motion and function may be appropriate after pain and spasm are relieved.

76. The answer is a. *(Braunwald, 15/e, pp 1987–1993.)* The clinical picture of a noninflammatory arthritis of weight-bearing joints is suggestive of degenerative joint disease, also called osteoarthritis. Crepitation over the involved joints is characteristic, as are bony enlargements of the DIP joints. In this overweight patient, weight reduction is the best method to decrease the risk of further degenerative changes. Aspirin or acetominophen can be used as symptomatic treatment, but do not affect the course of the disease. Calcium supplementation may be relevant to associated osteoporosis, but not to the osteoarthritis. Oral prednisone would be contraindicated; intraarticular corticosteroid injections may be given two to three times per year for symptom reduction. Knee replacement is the treatment of last resort, usually when pain occurs around the clock and symptoms are not controlled by medical regimens.

77. The answer is b. *(Braunwald, 15/e, pp 1949–1955.)* Insidious back pain occurring in a young male that improves with exercise suggests one of the spondyloarthropathies—ankylosing spondylitis, Reiter syndrome, psoriatic arthritis, or enteropathic arthritis. Ankylosing spondylitis is most likely in this patient. Acute lumbosacral strain would not be relieved by exercise or worsened by rest. The prognosis in ankylosing spondylitis is generally very good, with only 6% dying of the disease itself. While pulmonary fibrosis and restrictive lung disease can occur, it is rarely a cause of death (cervical fracture, heart block, and amyloidosis are leading causes of death due to ankylosing spondylitis). Rheumatoid factor is negative in all the spondyloarthropathies. Crohn's disease can cause an enteropathic arthritis, but this diagnosis is unlikely without gastrointestinal symptoms.

78. The answer is a. *(Braunwald, 15/e, pp 1922–1927.)* The combination of fever, malar rash, and arthritis suggests systemic lupus erythematosus, and the patient's thrombocytopenia, leukopenia, and positive antibody to native DNA provide more than four criteria for a definitive diagnosis. Other criteria for the diagnosis of lupus include discoid rash, photosensitivity, oral ulcers, serositis, renal disorders (proteinuria or cellular casts), and neurologic disorder (seizures). High-dose corticosteroids would therefore be indicated for any life-threatening complication of lupus such as described in item a. Patients with SLE have an unpredictable course. Few patients develop all signs or symptoms. Neuropsychiatric disease occurs at some time in about half of all SLE patients, and Raynaud's phenomenon in about 25%. Pregnancy is relatively safe in women with SLE who have controlled disease and are on less than 10 mg of prednisone.

79. The answer is b. (*Braunwald, 15/e, pp 1937–1945.*) The symptoms of Raynaud's phenomenon, arthralgia, and dysphagia point toward the diagnosis of scleroderma. Scleroderma or systemic sclerosis is characterized by a systemic vasculopathy of small and medium-sized vessels, excessive collagen deposition in tissues, and an abnormal immune system. It is an uncommon multisystem disease affecting women more than men. There are two variants of scleroderma—a benign type called the CREST syndrome and a more severe diffuse disease. Antinucleolar antibody occurs in only 20 to 30% of patients with the disease, but a positive test is highly specific. Cardiac involvement may occur, and an ECG could show heart block or pericardial involvement. Renal failure can develop insidiously. Rheumatoid factor is nonspecific and present in 20% of patients with scleroderma.

80. The answer is c. (*Stobo, 23/e, p 230.*) Reiter syndrome is a reactive polyarthritis that develops several weeks after an infection such as non-gonococcal urethritis or gastrointestinal infection caused by *Yersinia enterocolitica, Campylobacter jejuni,* or *Salmonella* or *Shigella* species. Reiter syndrome is characterized as a triad of oligoarticular arthritis, conjunctivitis, and urethritis. The disease is most common among young men and is associated with the HLA-B27 locus. A circinate balanitis is painless and occurs in 25 to 40% of patients. Other clinical features may include waxy papules on the palms and soles called keratoderma blenorrhagicum, spondylitis, myocarditis, and thrombophlebitis. ANA and rheumatoid factor are usually negative. Gonorrhea can precipitate Reiter syndrome, but patients with the disease are culture negative.

81. The answer is c. *(Braunwald, 15/e, pp 123, 1963.)* Unilateral headache and visual loss in this elderly patient with polymyalgia rheumatica (PMR) symptoms lead to a clinical diagnosis of temporal arteritis. The erythrocyte sedimentation rate is high in almost all of these patients. Skull x-ray and CT scan would be normal. Carotid disease would not be expected. Temporal arteritis occurs most commonly in patients over the age of 55 and is highly associated with polymyalgia rheumatica. About 25% of patients with PMR have some features of giant cell arteritis. Thus, older patients who complain of diffuse myalgias and joint stiffness, particularly of the shoulders and hips, should be evaluated for PMR with ESR. Sudden visual loss in such a patient makes temporal arteritis an important diagnosis to make quickly.

82. The answer is a. *(Braunwald, 15/e, p 1964.)* Biopsy results should not delay corticosteroid therapy. Biopsies may show vasculitis even after 14 days of glucocorticoid therapy. Delay risks permanent loss of sight. Once an episode of loss of vision occurs, workup must proceed as quickly as possible. Treatment for temporal arteritis requires relatively high doses of steroids, beginning with prednisone at 40 to 60 mg for about 1 month. The treatment for polymyalgia rheumatica requires much lower doses of steroids.

83. The answer is c. *(Braunwald, 15/e, pp 1995–1996.)* The acute mono-articular arthritis in association with linear calcification of the cartilage of the knee suggests the diagnosis of pseudogout, also called calcium pyro-phosphate dihydrate deposition disease. The disease resembles gout. Positive birefringent crystals (looking blue when parallel to the axis of the red compensator on a polarizing microscope) can be demonstrated in joint fluid. Serum uric acid and calcium levels are normal, as is the rheumatoid factor. Pseudogout is about half as common as gout but becomes more common after age 65. Calcium pyrophosphate dihydrate deposition disease is diagnosed in symptomatic patients by characteristic x-ray findings or crystals in synovial fluid. The disease is treated with NSAIDs or colchicine. Linear calcifications or chondrocalcinosis are often found in the joints of elderly patients who do not have symptomatic joint problems; such patients do not require treatment.

84. The answer is b. *(Braunwald, 15/e, pp 1995–1996.)* Pseudogout may be associated with hemochromatosis. Since the patient has a history of diabetes mellitus and cardiomyopathy, this process must be considered. Serum iron saturation should be measured. Pseudogout has also been associated with hyperparathyroidism. A familial form of the disease has been localized to chromosomes 8q and 5p.

85. The answer is a. (*Braunwald, 15/e, pp 2010–2011.*) The patient's multiple trigger points, associated sleep disturbance, and lack of joint or muscle findings make fibromyalgia a possible diagnosis. The diagnosis hinges on the multiple tender points. CBC and ESR are characteristically normal. Tricyclic antidepressants restore sleep; aspirin and other anti-inflammatory drugs are not helpful. Biofeedback and exercise programs have been partially successful. The clavicle, medial malleolus, and forehead are never trigger points for the process.

86. The answer is c. (*Braunwald, 15/e, p 1986.*) Hip pain may result from fracture, bursitis, enthesitis, sacroiliac pain, sciatica, or pain referred from the lumbosacral spine. A film of the right hip is mandatory in this patient. Fracture of the hip must be ruled out, particularly in a woman with mental status abnormalities, who may be prone to falls. Elderly women with osteoporosis are most prone to hip fracture.

87–90. The answers are 87-f, 88-c, 89-a, 90-b. (*Braunwald, 15/e, pp 123, 1949–1952, 1956, 1958–1959.*) Behçet syndrome is a multisystem disorder that usually presents with recurrent oral and genital ulcers. One-fourth of patients develop superficial or deep vein thrombophlebitis. Iritis, uveitis, and nondeforming arthritis may also occur.

The 50-year-old drug abuser also has a multisystem disease, including systemic complaints, hypertension, skin lesions, neuropathy, and an abnormal urine sediment. This complex suggests a vasculitis, particularly polyarteritis nodosa. Twenty to 30% of patients have hepatitis B antigenemia. The disease is a necrotizing vasculitis of small and medium muscular arteries. The pathology of the kidney includes an arteritis and, in some cases, a glomerulitis. Nodular skin lesions show vasculitis on biopsy.

The 19-year-old with low back pain, morning stiffness, and eye pain has complaints that suggest ankylosing spondylitis. This is an inflammatory disorder that affects the axial skeleton. It is an autoimmune disorder that has a close association with HLA-B27 histocompatibility antigen. Anterior uveitis is the most common extraarticular complaint. Aortic regurgitation occurs in a few percent of patients.

The elderly male presents with nonspecific joint complaints typical of polymyalgia rheumatica. The high erythrocyte sedimentation rate is characteristic. The transient loss of vision suggests concomitant temporal arteritis, an important association seen particularly in older patients.

91. The answer is c. (*Braunwald, 15/e, pp 369, 1932.*) Felty syndrome consists of a triad of rheumatoid arthritis, splenomegaly, and leukopenia. In contrast to the lymphopenia observed in patients who have systemic lupus erythematosus, the leukopenia of Felty syndrome is related to a reduction in the number of circulating polymorphonuclear leukocytes. The mechanism of the granulocytopenia is poorly understood. Felty syndrome tends to occur in people who have had active rheumatoid arthritis for a prolonged period. These patients commonly have other systemic features of rheumatoid disease such as nodules, skin ulcerations, the sicca complex, peripheral sensory and motor neuropathy, and arteritic lesions.

92–96. The answers are 92-a, 93-c, 94-d, 95-b, 96-b. (*Braunwald, 15/e, pp 1935–1936.*) Drugs used in the treatment of rheumatoid arthritis are broadly classified as anti-inflammatory or disease-modifying agents. Aspirin, a nonsteroidal anti-inflammatory agent that inhibits prostaglandin synthesis, is a commonly used first-line drug. The most frequent side effect is gastrointestinal distress. Gold therapy is still used in some patients with rheumatoid arthritis, especially in those who have not tolerated methotrexate. However, side effects are significant and include a dermatitis that may lead to exfoliative dermatitis if treatment is not discontinued, stomatitis, the nephrotic syndrome, and bone marrow suppression. Patients' response to gold may be only temporary. Low-dose prednisone may be very useful in controlling an acute flare-up of arthritis or in controlling the disease while waiting for a remittive agent to begin working. However, prednisone has significant toxicity, including causing osteoporosis. The most significant side effect of chloroquine is deposition of the drug in the pigmented layer of the retina. Irreversible retinal degeneration may develop, and this has limited the use of this drug. Hydroxychloroquine (Plaquenil) is less frequently associated with retinopathy. Ophthalmic examinations are required every 6 months during therapy.

97–101. The answers are 97-b, 98-d, 99-a, 100-c, 101-e. *(Braunwald,
15/e, pp 1956–1968.)* Wegener's granulomatosis is a granulomatous vasculitis of small arteries and veins that affects the lungs, sinuses, nasopharynx,
and kidneys, where it causes a focal and segmental glomerulonephritis.
Other organs can also be damaged, including the skin, eyes, and nervous
system. Most patients with the disease develop antibodies to certain proteins in the cytoplasm of neutrophils called antineutrophil cytoplasmic
antibodies (ANCA).

Elderly people may have extensive atherosclerosis. Especially after an
endovascular procedure (such as vascular catheterization, grafting, or
repair), some of the atheromatous material may embolize, usually to the skin,
kidneys, or brain. This material is capable of fixing complement and thus
causing vascular damage. The skin lesions—ecchymoses and necrosis—look
much like vasculitis. Differentiation between cholesterol embolization and
idiopathic vasculitis is important, since not only is the former not steroid-
sensitive, but there have been reports of increasing damage after the institution of steroid therapy.

Polyarteritis nodosa is a multisystem necrotizing vasculitis that, prior
to the use of steroids and cyclophosphamide, was uniformly fatal. In 30%
of patients, antecedent hepatitis B virus infection can be demonstrated;
immune complexes containing the virus have been found in such patients
and are likely pathogenetic.

Giant cell arteritis, also referred to as temporal arteritis or cranial
arteritis, is a disease of elderly patients that classically affects the temporal
arteries. Giant cell arteritis, named for the presence of giant cells and gran-
ulomata that disrupt the internal elastica of the vessel, may present with
headache, anemia, a high ESR (although a normal ESR does not rule out
the diagnosis), and occasionally a syndrome known as polymyalgia
rheumatica. This includes stiffness, aching, and tenderness of the proximal
muscles. These patients describe weakness of the hip and shoulder girdles,
but there is no objective weakness of the muscles, and the muscle enzymes
are normal. Giant cell arteritis usually responds to steroid therapy with 40
to 60 mg/d of prednisone; polymyalgia rheumatica typically responds to
low-dose prednisone at 10 to 15 mg/d.

Takayasu's arteritis is a granulomatous inflammation of the aorta and
its main branches. Symptoms are due to local vascular occlusion. Aortic
regurgitation; systemic and pulmonary hypertension; and general symp-

toms of arthralgia, fatigue, malaise, anorexia, and weight loss may occur. Surgery may be necessary to correct occlusive lesions.

102. The answer is c. (Braunwald, 15/e, pp 123, 1980, 2010–2011.) The signs and symptoms described suggest fibromyalgia. Fibromyalgia is a very common disorder, particularly in middle-aged women, characterized by diffuse musculoskeletal pain, fatigability, and nonrestorative sleep. The disease is now better defined by physical exam that shows specific tender points. The American College of Rheumatology has established diagnostic criteria for the disease, which include a history of widespread pain in association with 11 of 18 specific tender point sites. In this patient with very characteristic signs and symptoms, the identification of 11 specific trigger points would be the best method of diagnosis. Polymyalgia rheumatica may sometimes be in the differential diagnosis. In this patient it would be particularly unlikely given the normal ESR. The disease process is distinct from dermatomyositis and muscle disease in that weakness is not prominent as compared to generalized pain. Fibromyalgia has been associated with symptoms of irritable bladder, headaches, and temporomandibular joint pain but not with classic symptoms of vasculitis. While patients may have psychological abnormalities, there is no specific psychiatric diagnosis associated with fibromyalgia. Patients may experience depression, anxiety, or hypochondriasis.

103. The answer is a. (Braunwald, 15/e, pp 1984–1986.) Carpal tunnel syndrome results from median nerve entrapment and is usually due to excessive use of the wrist. The process has been associated with thickening of connective tissue as in acromegaly, or with deposition of amyloid. It also occurs in hypothyroidism, rheumatoid arthritis, and diabetes mellitus. As in this patient, numbness occurs in the distribution of the median nerve. Later in the process, atrophy of the abductor pollicis brevis becomes apparent. The Tinel sign (parasthesia induced in the median nerve distribution by a reflex hammer hitting on the volar aspect of the wrist) is very characteristic. De Quervain's tenosynovitis causes focal wrist pain on the radial aspect of the hand and is due to inflammation of the tendon sheath of the abductor pollicis longus. It should not produce a postive Tinel sign. Amyotrophic lateral sclerosis may present with distal muscle weakness that is diffuse and not focal. Diffuse atrophy and muscle fasiculations would be prominent. Rheumatoid arthritis would not produce these symptoms unless inflammation of the wrist was causing median nerve entrapment in the carpal tunnel.

Pulmonary Disease

Questions

DIRECTIONS: Each item below contains a question or incomplete statement followed by suggested responses. Select the **one best** response to each question.

104. A 50-year-old patient with long-standing chronic obstructive lung disease develops the insidious onset of aching in the distal extremities, particularly the wrists bilaterally. There is a 10-lb weight loss. The skin over the wrists is warm and erythematous. There is bilateral clubbing. Plain film is read as periosteal thickening, possible osteomyelitis. You should

a. Start ciprofloxacin
b. Obtain chest x-ray
c. Aspirate both wrists
d. Begin gold therapy

105. A patient with low-grade fever and weight loss has poor excursion on the right side of the chest with decreased fremitus, flatness to percussion, and decreased breath sounds all on the right. The trachea is deviated to the left. The most likely diagnosis is

a. Pneumothorax
b. Pleural effusion
c. Consolidated pneumonia
d. Atelectasis

106. A 60-year-old female with a history of urinary tract infection, steroid-dependent chronic obstructive lung disease, and asthma presents with bilateral infiltrates and an eosinophil count of 15%. The least likely diagnosis is

a. Bronchopulmonary aspergillosis
b. Hypersensitivity pneumonitis
c. *Strongyloides* hyperinfection syndrome
d. Drug effect of nitrofurantoin

107. A 40-year-old alcoholic develops cough and fever. Chest x-ray shows an air-fluid level in the superior segment of the right lower lobe. The most likely etiologic agent is

a. *Streptococcus pneumoniae*
b. *Haemophilus influenzae*
c. *Legionella*
d. Anaerobes

DIRECTIONS: Each group of questions below consists of lettered options followed by a set of numbered items. For each numbered item, select the **one** lettered option with which it is **most** closely associated. Each lettered option may be used once, more than once, or not at all.

Items 108–112

Match the disease entity with the type of pleural effusion.

a. pH less than 7.0
b. Right-sided effusion, protein 2.5 g/dL
c. Pleural fluid glucose less than 15 mg/dL
d. Exudate, 100% lymphocytes
e. Bloody effusion
f. Milky appearance
g. Low cholesterol

108. Congestive heart failure **(CHOOSE 1 EFFUSION)**

109. Tuberculosis **(CHOOSE 1 EFFUSION)**

110. Empyema **(CHOOSE 1 EFFUSION)**

111. Rheumatoid arthritis **(CHOOSE 1 EFFUSION)**

112. Mesothelioma **(CHOOSE 1 EFFUSION)**

Items 113–116

Match the chest x-ray letter with the most likely clinical description.

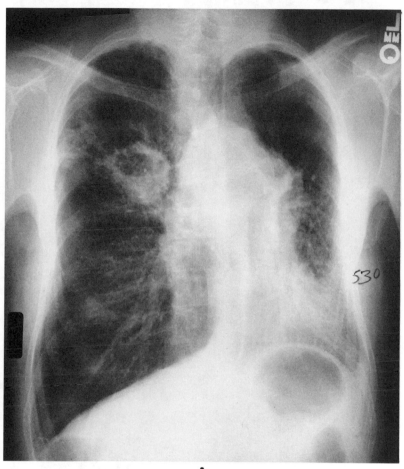

A

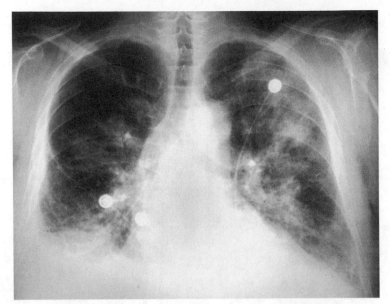

B

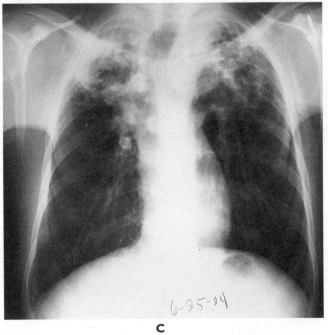

C

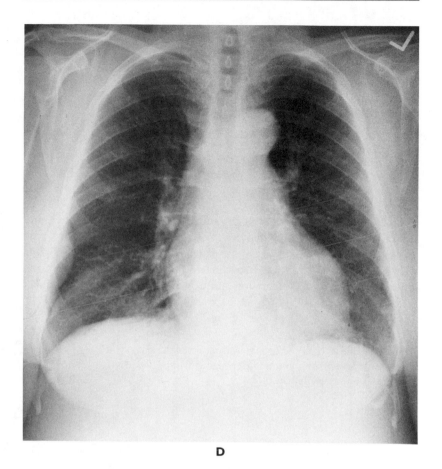

D

113. Fever, shaking chills; sputum Gram stain showing gram-positive cocci in clusters **(CHOOSE 1 X-RAY)**

114. Shortness of breath, awakens gasping for breath at night **(CHOOSE 1 X-RAY)**

115. Fever, night sweats for 1 year **(CHOOSE 1 X-RAY)**

116. Long-standing hypertension **(CHOOSE 1 X-RAY)**

117. A 30-year-old male is admitted to the hospital after a motorcycle accident that resulted in a fracture of the right femur. The fracture is managed with traction. Three days later the patient becomes confused and tachypneic. A petechial rash is noted over the chest. Lungs are clear to auscultation. Arterial blood gases show PO_2 of 50, PCO_2 of 28, and pH of 7.49. The most likely diagnosis is

a. Unilateral pulmonary edema
b. Hematoma of the chest
c. Fat embolism
d. Pulmonary embolism
e. Early *Staphylococcus aureus* pneumonia

118. A 70-year-old patient with chronic obstructive lung disease requires 2 L of nasal O_2 to treat his hypoxia, which is sometimes associated with angina. While receiving nasal O_2, the patient develops pleuritic chest pain, fever, and purulent sputum. He becomes stuporous and develops a respiratory acidosis with CO_2 retention and worsening hypoxia. The treatment of choice is

a. Stop oxygen
b. Begin medroxyprogesterone
c. Intubate the trachea and begin mechanical ventilation
d. Observe patient 24 hours before changing therapy
e. Begin sodium bicarbonate

119. A 34-year-old black female presents to your office with symptoms of cough, dyspnea, and lymphadenopathy. Physical exam shows cervical adenopathy and hepatomegaly. Her chest radiograph is shown below. How should you pursue diagnosis?

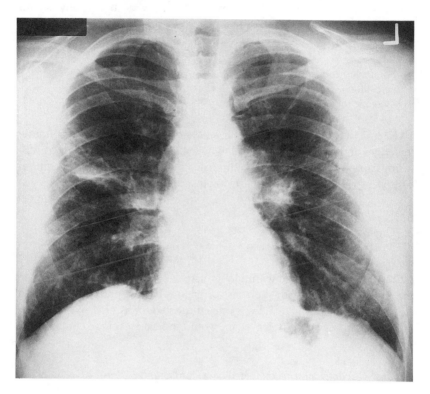

a. Open lung biopsy
b. Liver biopsy
c. Bronchoscopy and transbronchial lung biopsy
d. Scalene node biopsy
e. Serum angiotensin converting enzyme (ACE) level

120. A 64-year-old woman is found to have a left-sided pleural effusion on chest x-ray. Analysis of the pleural fluid reveals a ratio of concentration of total protein in pleural fluid to serum of 0.38, a lactate dehydrogenase (LDH) level of 125 IU, and a ratio of LDH concentration in pleural fluid to serum of 0.46. Which of the following disorders is most likely in this patient?

a. Uremia
b. Congestive heart failure
c. Pulmonary embolism
d. Sarcoidosis
e. Systemic lupus erythematosus

121. A 25-year-old male cigarette smoker has a history of respiratory infections and has also been found to have hematuria. A high value for diffusing capacity is noted during pulmonary function testing. This finding is consistent with which of the following disorders?

a. Anemia
b. Cystic fibrosis
c. Emphysema
d. Intrapulmonary hemorrhage

122. A 25-year-old male with a long history of severe asthma presents to the emergency room with shortness of breath. He has previously required admission to the hospital and was once intubated for asthma. Which of the following findings on physical exam would indicate a benign course?

a. Silent chest
b. Hypercapnia
c. Thoracoabdominal paradox (paradoxical respiration)
d. Pulsus paradoxus of 5 mmHg
e. Altered mental status

123. A 40-year-old man without a significant past medical history comes to the emergency room with a 3-day history of fever and shaking chills; a 15-minute episode of rigor; nonproductive cough; anorexia; and the development of right-sided pleuritic chest pain and shortness of breath over the last 12 hours. A chest x-ray reveals a consolidated right middle lobe infiltrate, and a CBC shows an elevated neutrophil count with many band forms present. Which of the following statements regarding pneumonia in this patient is correct?

a. Sputum culture is more helpful than sputum Gram stain in choosing empiric antibiotic therapy
b. If the Gram stain revealed numerous gram-positive diplococci, numerous white blood cells, and few epithelial cells, *Streptococcus pneumoniae* would be the most likely diagnosis
c. Although *S. pneumoniae* is the agent most likely to be the cause of this patient's pneumonia, this diagnosis would be very unlikely if blood cultures were negative
d. The absence of rigors would rule out a diagnosis of pneumococcal pneumonia
e. Penicillin is the drug of choice in all cases of pneumococcal pneumonia

Items 124–125

124. A 57-year-old man develops acute shortness of breath shortly after a 12-hour automobile ride. The patient consults his internist, and findings on physical examination are normal except for tachypnea and tachycardia. An electrocardiogram reveals sinus tachycardia but is otherwise normal. Which of the following is correct?

a. A definitive diagnosis can be made by history alone
b. The patient should be admitted to the hospital, and, if there is no contraindication to anticoagulation, intravenous heparin should be started pending further testing
c. Normal findings on examination of the lower extremities are extremely unusual in this clinical setting
d. Early treatment has little effect on overall mortality

125. The most important next step in the diagnosis of this patient is

a. Pulmonary angiogram
b. Ventilation-perfusion scan
c. D-dimer assay
d. Venous ultrasound

126. An anxious young woman who is taking birth control pills presents to the emergency room with shortness of breath. The absence of which of the following would make the diagnosis of pulmonary embolus unlikely?

a. Wheezing
b. Pleuritic chest pain
c. Tachypnea
d. Hemoptysis
e. Right-sided S_3 heart sound

127. A 65-year-old male with mild congestive heart failure is to receive total hip replacement. He has no other underlying diseases and no history of hypertension, recent surgery, or bleeding disorder. The best approach to prevention of pulmonary embolus in this patient is

a. Aspirin 75 mg/d
b. Aspirin 325 mg/d
c. Warfarin with INR of 2 to 3
d. Early ambulation

128. A 30-year-old athlete with asthma is also a cigarette smoker. Which of the following is characteristic of asthma but not other obstructive lung disease?

a. Hyperinflation is present on chest x-ray
b. Airway obstruction is reversible
c. Hypoxia occurs as a consequence of ventilation-perfusion mismatch
d. The FEV_1/FVC ratio is reduced
e. Exacerbation often occurs as a result of an upper respiratory tract infection

Items 129–133

For each clinical situation, select the arterial blood gas and pH values with which it is most likely to be associated.

a. pH 7.50, Po_2 75, Pco_2 28
b. pH 7.15, Po_2 78, Pco_2 92
c. pH 7.06, Po_2 36, Pco_2 95
d. pH 7.06, Po_2 108, Pco_2 13
e. pH 7.39, Po_2 48, Pco_2 54

129. A 30-year-old obese female bus driver develops sudden pleuritic left-sided chest pain and dyspnea. **(CHOOSE 1 SET OF VALUES)**

130. A 60-year-old heavy smoker has severe chronic bronchitis and peripheral edema and cyanosis. **(CHOOSE 1 SET OF VALUES)**

131. A 22-year-old drug-addicted man is brought to the emergency room by friends who were unable to awaken him. **(CHOOSE 1 SET OF VALUES)**

132. A 62-year-old man who has chronic bronchitis and chest pain is given oxygen via mask in the ambulance en route to the hospital and becomes lethargic in the emergency room. **(CHOOSE 1 SET OF VALUES)**

133. A 20-year-old man with diabetes mellitus comes to the emergency room with diffuse abdominal pain, tachypnea, and fever. **(CHOOSE 1 SET OF VALUES)**

Items 134–138

For each set of findings below, select the disease with which it is most likely to be associated.

a. Asthma
b. Rheumatoid arthritis
c. α_1 antitrypsin deficiency
d. Cystic fibrosis
e. Sarcoidosis

134. Low levels of glucose in pleural effusions **(SELECT 1 DISEASE)**

135. Bronchiectasis and severe hemoptysis as frequent complications of clinical course **(SELECT 1 DISEASE)**

136. Presence of the mucoid strain of *Pseudomonas aeruginosa* **(SELECT 1 DISEASE)**

137. Development of severe liver disease that is usually associated with, but may be independent of, lung disease **(SELECT 1 DISEASE)**

138. Development of symptoms after ingestion of tartrazine yellow or aspirin **(SELECT 1 DISEASE)**

139. A 60-year-old male has had a chronic cough for over 5 years with clear sputum production. He has smoked one pack of cigarettes per day for 20 years and continues to do so. X-ray of the chest shows hyperinflation without infiltrates. Arterial blood gases show a pH of 7.38, P_{CO_2} of 40 mmHg, and P_{O_2} of 65 mmHg. Spirometry shows an FEV_1/FVC of 65%. The most important treatment modality for this patient is

a. Oral corticosteroids
b. Home oxygen
c. Broad-spectrum antibiotics
d. Smoking cessation program

140. A 50-year-old male with emphysema and a chest x-ray that has shown apical blebs develops the sudden onset of shortness of breath and left-sided pleuritic chest pain. Pneumothorax is suspected. Physical examination findings that would confirm the diagnosis are

a. Localized wheezes at the left base
b. Hyperresonance of the left chest with decreased breath sounds
c. Increased tactile fremitus on the left side
d. Decreased breath sounds on the left side with deviation of the trachea to the left

141. A 30-year-old paraplegic male has a long history of urinary tract infection secondary to an indwelling Foley catheter. He develops fever and hypotension requiring hospitalization, fluid therapy, and intravenous antibiotics. He improves, but over 1 week becomes increasingly short of breath and tachypneic. He develops frothy sputum, diffuse rales, and diffuse alveolar infiltrates. There is no fever, jugular venous distention, S_3 gallop, or peripheral or sacral edema. The best approach to a definitive diagnosis in this patient is

a. Blood cultures
b. CT scan of the chest
c. Pulmonary capillary wedge pressure
d. Ventilation-perfusion scan

142. A 35-year-old female complains of slowly progressive dyspnea. Her history is otherwise unremarkable, and there is no cough, sputum production, pleuritic chest pain, or thrombophlebitis. She has taken appetite suppressants at different times. On physical exam, there is jugular venous distention, a palpable right ventricular lift, and a loud P_2 heart sound. Chest x-ray shows clear lung fields. ECG shows right axis deviation. A perfusion lung scan is normal with no segmental deficits. The most likely diagnosis in this patient is

a. Primary pulmonary hypertension
b. Recurrent pulmonary emboli
c. Cardiac shunt
d. Interstitial lung disease

143. In the evaluation of this patient, cardiac catheterization confirms the diagnosis. The next step in the management of the patient is

a. Acute drug testing with short-acting pulmonary vasodilators
b. High-dose nifedipine
c. Intravenous prostacyclin
d. Lung transplantation

144. A 60-year-old obese male complains of excessive daytime sleepiness. He has been in good health except for mild hypertension. He drinks alcohol in moderation. The patient's wife states that he snores at night and awakens frequently. Examination of the oropharynx is normal. Which of the following studies is most appropriate?

a. EEG to assess stage sleep patterns
b. Ventilation pattern to detect apnea
c. Arterial O_2 saturation
d. Polysomnography to include all of the above

145. The patient above is found to have recurrent episodes of arterial desaturation—about 15 events per hour—with evidence of obstructive apnea. The treatment of choice for this patient is

a. Nasal continuous positive airway pressure
b. Uvulopalatopharyngoplasty
c. Weight reduction
d. Tracheostomy

Pulmonary Disease

Answers

104. The answer is b. *(Braunwald, 15/e, pp 2008–2010.)* The clinical picture suggests hypertrophic osteoarthropathy. This process, the pathogenesis of which is unknown, is characterized by clubbing of digits, periosteal new bone formation, and arthritis. Hypertrophic osteoarthropathy is associated with intrathoracic malignancy, suppurative lung disease, and congenital heart problems. Treatment is directed at the underlying disease process. While x-rays may suggest osteomyelitis, the process is usually bilateral and easily distinguishable from osteomyelitis. The first step in evaluation of this patient is to obtain a chest x-ray looking for lung infection and carcinoma.

105. The answer is b. *(Braunwald, 15/e, pp 1444–1445.)* The diagnosis in this patient is suggested by the physical exam findings. The findings of poor excursion, flatness of percussion, and decreased fremitus on the right side are all consistent with a right-sided pleural effusion. A large right-sided effusion may shift the trachea to the left. Histoplasmosis would be one possible cause of such an effusion. A pneumothorax should result in hyperresonance of the affected side. Atelectasis on the right side would shift the trachea to the right. A consolidated pneumonia would characteristically result in increased fremitus, flatness to percussion, and bronchial breath sounds, and would not cause tracheal deviation.

106. The answer is b. *(Braunwald, 15/e, pp 1460, 1465.)* This 60-year-old woman has peripheral eosinophilia in association with pulmonary infiltrates. The differential diagnosis for eosinophilic pneumonia includes allergic bronchopulmonary aspergillosis, parasitic infections, drug reactions, and a category of idiopathic disease. Nitrofurdantoin and sulfonamides are among the drugs most likely to cause eosinophilic pneumonia. Hypersensitivity pneumonitis may cause bilateral infiltrates, but does not of itself cause eosinophilia.

107. The answer is d. *(Braunwald, 15/e, p 1478.)* Of the organisms listed, only anaerobic infection is likely to cause a necrotizing process. Type III pneumococci have been reported to cause cavitary disease, but this is unusual. The location of the infiltrate suggests aspiration, also making anaerobic infection most likely. The superior segment of the right lower lobe is the one most likely to develop an aspiration pneumonia.

108–112. The answers are 108-b, 109-d, 110-a, 111-c, 112-e. (*Braunwald, 15/e, pp 1513–1515.*) The first step in determining the cause of a pleural effusion is to categorize it as either a transudate or exudate. Transudative effusions occur when factors alter the formation or absorption of pleural fluid; exudative effusions occur when local factors produce an inflammatory process. Exudative effusions have one of the following characteristics: pleural fluid protein–to–serum protein ratio greater than 0.5, pleural fluid LDH–to–serum LDH ratio greater than 0.6, or pleural fluid LDH more than two-thirds the normal upper limit for serum. Congestive heart failure usually produces a right-sided pleural effusion. Of all the disease processes listed, it is the only one that usually results in a transudative effusion.

Tuberculosis causes a hypersensitivity reaction to tuberculous protein in the pleural fluid. It produces an exudative effusion with small lymphocytes. The diagnosis is now established by demonstrating high levels of TB markers such as adenosine deaminase or positive PCR for tuberculous DNA.

Empyema may be defined by the very low pH value. It is an exudative effusion with a polymorphonuclear leukocyte predominance. A drainage procedure is usually necessary when the pleural fluid pH is below 7.20, when there is gross pus, or when the fluid shows a positive gram stain or culture.

Rheumatoid effusions are often exudative and may be lymphocytic, but they are best characterized by their very low glucose levels. Pleural fluid glucose levels below 60 mg/dL also occur in malignancy and bacterial infections.

Mesotheliomas are primary tumors that arise from mesothelial cells that line the pleural cavity. They produce a very bloody effusion. Thoracoscopy or open pleural biopsy are often necessary to make a definitive diagnosis.

113–116. The answers are 113-a, 114-b, 115-c, 116-d. (*Braunwald, 15/e, pp 1030, 1323, 1477–1478.*) The patient with fever, shaking chills, and a Gram stain showing gram-positive cocci in clusters has *Staphylococcus* *aureus* pneumonia. Chest x-ray A shows a necrotizing pneumonia characteristic of this infection. Cavities develop in association with lung infection when necrotic lung tissue is discharged into airways. Cavities greater than 2 cm are described as lung abscesses.

The patient with shortness of breath and paroxysmal nocturnal dyspnea might have chest x-ray B, which shows signs of congestive heart failure including cardiomegaly, bilateral infiltrates, and cephalization. When there has been long-standing venous hypertension, upper lobe vessels become more prominent due to redistribution of pulmonary blood flow. When pulmonary edema becomes severe, fluid extends out from the hila in a batwing distribution.

Chest x-ray C is best matched with the patient who has fever and night sweats. This x-ray shows characteristic changes of tuberculosis, including extensive apical and upper lobe scarring. When the lung is involved with tuberculosis, the range of abnormalities is broad. Cavitary infiltrates in the posterior apical segments are very common. Mass lesions, interstitial infiltrates, and noncavitary infiltrates also occur.

The patient with long-standing hypertension shows chest x-ray evidence for left ventricular hypertrophy. The cardiac silhouette is enlarged and takes on a boot-shaped configuration, as seen in chest x-ray D.

117. The answer is c. (*Braunwald, 15/e, p 329.*) Because the clinical signs of neurologic deterioration and a petechial rash have occurred in the setting of fracture and hypoxia, fat embolism is the most likely diagnosis. This process occurs when neutral fat is introduced into the venous circulation after bone trauma or fracture. The latent period is 12 to 36 hours, usually earlier than a pulmonary embolus would occur after trauma.

118. The answer is c. (*Braunwald, 15/e, p 1525.*) When stupor and coma supervene in CO_2 retention, fatal arrhythmias, seizures, and death are likely to follow. Stopping oxygen is the worst course of action, as it will exacerbate life-threatening hypoxia. Intubation is the only good alternative. Bicarbonate plays no role in this acidosis, which is respiratory and caused by hypoventilation.

119. The answer is c. (*Braunwald, 15/e, pp 1969–1974.*) Sarcoidosis is a systemic illness of unknown etiology. Many patients have respiratory symptoms, including cough and dyspnea. Hilar and peripheral lymphadenopathy is common, and 20 to 30% of patients have hepatomegaly. The chest x-ray shows symmetrical hilar lymphadenopathy. The diagnostic method of choice is transbronchial biopsy, which will show a mononuclear cell granulomatous inflammatory process. While liver and scalene node biopsies are often positive, noncaseating granulomas are so frequent in these sites that they are not considered acceptable for primary diagnosis. ACE levels are elevated in two-thirds of patients, but false-positive values are common in other granulomatous disease processes.

120. The answer is b. (*Braunwald, 15/e, p 1513.*) Classifying a pleural effusion as either a transudate or an exudate is useful in identifying the underlying disorder. Pleural fluid is exudative if it has any one of the following three properties: a ratio of concentration of total protein in pleural fluid to serum greater than 0.5, an absolute value of LDH greater than 200 IU, or a ratio of LDH concentration in pleural fluid to serum greater than 0.6. Causes of exudative effusions include malignancy, pulmonary embolism, pneumonia, tuberculosis, abdominal disease, collagen vascular diseases, uremia, Dressler syndrome, and chylothorax. Exudative effusions may also be drug-induced. If none of the aforementioned properties are met, the effusion is a transudate. Differential diagnosis includes congestive heart failure, nephrotic syndrome, cirrhosis, Meigs syndrome (benign ovarian neoplasm with effusion), and hydronephrosis.

121. The answer is d. (*Braunwald, 15/e, pp 1450–1451.*) Carbon monoxide (CO) diffusing capacity provides an estimate of the rate at which oxygen moves by diffusion from alveolar gas to combine with hemoglobin in the red blood cells. It is interpreted as an index of the surface area engaged in alveolar-capillary diffusion. Measurement of diffusing capacity of the lung is done by having the person inspire a low concentration of carbon monoxide. The rate of uptake of the gas by the blood is calculated from the difference between the inspired and expired concentrations. The test can be performed during a single 10-second breath holding or during 1 minute of steady-state breathing. The diffusing capacity is defined as the amount of carbon monoxide transferred per minute per millimeter of mercury of driving pressure and correlates with oxygen transport from the alveolus into the capillaries. Primary parenchymal disorders, anemia, and removal of lung tissue decrease the diffusing capacity. Conversely, polycythemia, congestive heart failure, and intrapulmonary hemorrhage tend to increase the value for diffusing capacity. In this patient, the possibility of Goodpasture syndrome would be considered.

122. The answer is d. (*Stobo, 23/e, p 143.*) It is extremely important to accurately determine the severity of an exacerbation of asthma, since the major cause of death from asthma is the underestimation of the severity of a particular episode by either the patient or the physician. Silent chest is a particularly ominous finding, because the airway constriction is so great that airflow is insufficient to generate wheezing. Hypercapnia and thoraco-abdominal paradox are almost always indicative of exhaustion and respiratory muscle failure or fatigue and generally need to be aggressively treated with mechanical ventilation. Altered mental status is frequently seen with severe hypoxia or hypercapnia, and ventilatory support is usually required. An increased pulsus paradoxus may also be a sign of severe asthma, as it increases with greater respiratory effort and generation of more negative intrathoracic pressures during inspiration. However, a pulsus paradoxus of up to 8 to 10 mmHg is considered normal; thus, a value of 5 mmHg would not be indicative of a severe episode of asthma.

123. The answer is b. (*Braunwald, 15/e, pp 1476–1482.*) Pneumonia is a common disorder and is a major cause of death, particularly in hospitalized elderly patients. Before choosing empiric therapy for presumed pneumonia, it is necessary to know the age of the patient, whether the infection is community-acquired or nosocomial, and whether there are any underlying debilitating illnesses. Community-acquired pneumonias in patients over the age of 35 are most likely due to *S. pneumoniae*, *Legionella* species (e.g., *pneumophila*), and *Haemophilus influenzae*. In the case outlined, the history is strongly consistent with pneumococcal pneumonia, manifested by a short prodrome, shaking chills with rigor, fever, chest pain, sparse sputum production associated with cough, and a consolidated lobar infiltrate on chest x-ray. The most reliable method of diagnosing pneumococcal pneumonia is seeing gram-positive diplococci on an adequate sputum (many white cells, few epithelial cells). Sputum culture is also important in the era of penicillin-resistant pneumococci, but is not helpful in initial diagnosis. Blood cultures are positive in only about 20% of patients, and, when positive, are indicative of a more severe case. Although rigors may suggest pneumococcal bacteremia, the absence of rigors does not rule out the diagnosis. About 25% of pneumococci in the United States are partially or completely resistant to penicillin due to chromosomal mutations resulting in penicillin-binding protein changes. Penicillin is no longer the regimen of choice for pneumococcal pneumonia pending the results of sensitivity testing. The fluoroquinolones or ceftriaxone are widely used as initial therapy for pneumococcal pneumonia.

124. The answer is b. *(Braunwald, 15/e, pp 1508–1512.)* The clinical situation described is characteristic of pulmonary embolic disease. In greater than 80% of cases, pulmonary emboli arise from thromboses in the deep venous circulation (DVTs) of the lower extremities. DVTs often begin in the calf, where they rarely if ever cause clinically significant pulmonary embolic disease. However, thromboses that begin below the knee frequently "grow," or propagate, above the knee; clots that dislodge from above the knee cause clinically significant pulmonary emboli, which, if untreated, cause mortality exceeding 80%. Interestingly, only about 50% of patients with DVT of the lower extremities have clinical findings of swelling, warmth, erythema, pain, or "cords." As long as the superficial venous system, which has connections with the deep venous system, remains patent, none of the classic clinical findings of DVT will occur, because blood will drain from the unobstructed superficial system. When a clot does dislodge from the deep venous system and travels into the pulmonary vasculature, the most common clinical findings are tachypnea and tachycardia; chest pain is less likely and is more indicative of concomitant pulmonary infarction. The ABG is usually abnormal, and a high percentage of patients exhibit hypoxia, hypocapnia, alkalosis, and a widening of the alveolar-arterial gradient. The ECG is frequently abnormal in pulmonary embolic disease. The most common finding is sinus tachycardia, but atrial fibrillation, pseudoinfarction in the inferior leads, and right and left axis deviation are also occasionally seen. Initial treatment for suspected pulmonary embolic disease includes prompt hospitalization and institution of intravenous heparin, provided there are no contraindications to anticoagulation. It is particularly important to make an early diagnosis of pulmonary embolus, as intervention can decrease the mortality rate from 25% to 5%.

125. The answer is b. *(Braunwald, 15/e, pp 1509–1511.)* Lung scanning is the principal imaging test for the diagnosis of pulmonary embolus. The diagnosis is very unlikely in patients with normal or near normal scans, and is highly likely in patients with high-probability scans. In patients with a high clinical index of suspicion for pulmonary embolus but low-probability scan, the diagnosis becomes more difficult, and pulmonary angiography may be indicated. About two-thirds of patients with pulmonary embolus have evidence of deep venous disease on venous ultrasound. Therefore, pulmonary embolus cannot be excluded by a normal study. The quantitative D-dimer enzyme-linked immunoabsorbent assay is positive in 90% of patients with pulmonary embolus in some studies. It has been used to rule out pulmonary embolus in patients with a low- or intermediate-probability scan.

126. The answer is c. (*Braunwald, 15/e, p 1509.*) While all of these signs and symptoms can occur in acute pulmonary embolus, tachypnea is by far the most common. Tachypnea occurs in more than 90% of patients with pulmonary embolus. Pleuritic chest pain occurs in about half of patients and is less common in the elderly and those with underlying heart disease. Hemoptysis and wheezing occur in less than half of patients. A right-sided S_3 is associated with large emboli that result in acute pulmonary hypertension.

127. The answer is c. (*Braunwald, 15/e, p 1512.*) Warfarin is the principal agent recommended for the prophylaxis of acute pulmonary embolus in patients who receive total hip replacement. Warfarin is started preoperatively, and the daily dose is adjusted to maintain an international normalized ratio (INR) of 2 to 2.5. Low-molecular-weight heparin given twice daily subcutaneously is also a recommended regimen. The value of aspirin in this setting is unclear. Early ambulation and elastic stockings are also important in preventing thromboembolism, but are not adequate in themselves in this high-risk situation.

128. The answer is b. (*Braunwald, 15/e, pp 1456–1460.*) Asthma is an incompletely understood inflammatory process that involves the lower airways and results in bronchoconstriction and excess production of mucus, which in turn lead to increased airway resistance and occasionally respiratory failure and death. During acute exacerbations of asthma, and in other obstructive lung diseases such as chronic obstructive pulmonary disease, hyperinflation may be present on chest x-ray. Hypoxia is common and usually a result of ventilation-perfusion mismatch. The FEV_1/FVC is reduced, and exacerbations are frequently precipitated by upper airway infections. Only in asthma is the airway obstruction reversible.

129–133. The answers are 129-a, 130-e, 131-c, 132-b, 133-d. *(Stobo, 23/e, pp 121–125, 155–158, 162–176.)* The blood gas values associated with pulmonary embolism may vary tremendously. The most consistent finding is acute respiratory alkalosis. It is important to note that hypoxemia, although frequently found, need not be present. In severe chronic lung disease, the presence of hypercapnia leads to a compensatory increase in serum bicarbonate. Thus, significant hypercapnia may be present with an arterial pH close to normal, but will never be completely corrected. Acute respiratory acidosis may occur secondary to respiratory depression after drug overdose. Hypoventilation is associated with hypoxia; hypercapnia; and severe, uncompensated acidosis. In the presence of long-standing lung disease, respiration may become regulated by hypoxia rather than by altered carbon dioxide tension and arterial pH, as in normal people. Thus, the unmonitored administration of oxygen may lead to respiratory suppression, as in the patient described in the question, that results in acute and chronic respiratory acidosis. Young patients with type 1 diabetes mellitus may present with rapid onset of diabetic ketoacidosis (DKA), usually secondary to a systemic infection. These patients usually are maximally ventilating, as indicated by a very low arterial P_{CO_2}; however, they remain acidotic secondary to the severe metabolic ketoacidosis associated with this process. In general, these patients are not hypoxic unless the underlying infection is pneumonia.

134–138. The answers are 134-b, 135-d, 136-d, 137-c, 138-a. *(Braunwald, 15/e, pp 1456–1459, 1489, 1932, 1969–1973.)* Asthma is predominantly an inflammatory lower airway process. Frequent triggers of airway inflammation, and thus asthma, include infection, inhaled allergens, and processes that cool or dry the airways, such as exercise and exposure to cold weather. In addition, certain chemicals, such as aspirin (but not sodium or magnesium salicylate) and tartrazine yellow, have been implicated in the development of bronchospasm in certain patients.

Pleural effusions are not unusual in patients with rheumatoid arthritis. A history of pleurodynia that would suggest an antecedent inflammatory pleuritis is not always obtained, but characteristically, the pleural fluid, which is sterile, will contain a high level of lactic dehydrogenase and a low glucose concentration. Other pulmonary phenomena associated with rheumatoid arthritis include diffuse interstitial fibrosis and the occurrence of individual or clustered nodules in the lung parenchyma.

The fatality rate for patients with cystic fibrosis is lower today than in previous years; the average life span of patients afflicted with this disease has been significantly increasing. Chronic lung infections, however, are almost universal. The most common and difficult to treat of such infections is caused by the mucoid strain of *Pseudomonas aeruginosa*. Chronic coughing is one of the major and most distressing problems of patients with cystic fibrosis. Liver disease, particularly biliary cirrhosis, may develop in these patients. Common pulmonary complications include bronchiectasis, severe hemoptysis, and allergic bronchopulmonary aspergillosis. The incidence of liver disease associated with a deficiency of α_1 antitrypsin is very high. Patients with liver disease secondary to α_1 antitrypsin deficiency usually, but not always, have accompanying panacinar emphysema.

Sarcoidosis is a nonspecific granulomatous disease of unknown etiology. Blacks and Mediterranean peoples appear to be predisposed. The most commonly involved organs—after the lungs—are the liver, eye, spleen, skin, and kidney. The most characteristic presentation is a patient with a nonproductive cough with bilateral hilar adenopathy on chest x-ray. Treatment with prednisone is usually reserved for patients with diminishing pulmonary function, evidenced by reduced diffusing capacity or reduced lung volumes; 70 to 80% of untreated, stable patients will spontaneously remit.

139. The answer is d. *(Braunwald, 15/e, pp 1495–1498.)* This patient's chronic cough, hyperinflated lung fields, abnormal pulmonary function tests, and smoking history are all consistent with chronic bronchitis. A smoking cessation program can decrease the rate of lung deterioration and is successful in as many as 40% of patients, particularly when the physician gives a strong antismoking message and uses both counseling and nicotine replacement. Continuous low-flow oxygen becomes beneficial when arterial oxygen concentration falls below 55 mmHg. Antibiotics are indicated only for acute exacerbations of chronic lung disease, which might present with fever, change in color of sputum, and increasing shortness of breath. Oral corticosteroids are helpful in some patients, but are reserved for those who have failed inhaled bronchodilator treatments.

140. The answer is b. *(Braunwald, 15/e, p 1515.)* The most characteristic findings of pneumothorax are hyperresonance and decreased breath sounds. A tension pneumothorax may displace the mediastinum to the unaffected side. Tactile fremitus would be decreased in the patient with a pneumothorax, but would be increased in conditions in which consolidation of the lung has developed.

141. The answer is c. *(Braunwald, 15/e, pp 1523–1526.)* Sepsis is the most important single cause of adult respiratory distress syndrome. Early in the course of ARDS, patients may appear stable without respiratory symptoms. Tachypnea, hypoxemia, and diffuse infiltrates gradually develop. It may be difficult to distinguish the process from cardiogenic pulmonary edema, especially in patients who have been given large quantities of fluid. This young patient with no evidence of volume overload would be strongly suspected of having ARDS. The pulmonary capillary wedge pressure would be normal or low in ARDS, but elevated in left ventricular failure. ARDS is a complication of sepsis, but blood cultures may or may not be positive. Neither CT of the chest nor ventilation-perfusion scan would be specific enough to help in diagnosis of ARDS.

142. The answer is a. *(Braunwald, 15/e, pp 1506–1508.)* Although a difficult diagnosis to make, primary pulmonary hypertension is the most likely diagnosis in this young woman who has used appetite suppressants. There has been a recent increase in primary pulmonary hypertension in the United States associated with fenfluramines. The predominant symptom is dyspnea, which is usually not apparent in the previously healthy young woman until the disease has advanced. When signs of pulmonary hypertension are apparent from physical findings, chest x-ray, or echocardiography, the diagnosis of recurrent pulmonary embolus must be ruled out. In this case, a normal perfusion lung scan makes pulmonary angiography unnecessary. Restrictive lung disease should be ruled out with pulmonary function testing. An echocardiogram will show right ventricular enlargement and a reduction in the left ventricle size consistent with right ventricular pressure overload.

143. The answer is a. *(Braunwald, 15/e, pp 1507–1508.)* In all patients in whom primary pulmonary hypertension is confirmed, acute drug testing with a pulmonary vasodilator is necessary to assess the extent of pulmonary vascular reactivity. Inhaled nitric oxide, intravenous adenosine, or intravenous prostacyclin have all been used. Patients who have a good response to the short-acting vasodilator are tried on a long-acting calcium channel antagonist under direct hemodynamic monitoring. Prostacyclin has been approved for patients who are functional class III or IV and have not responded to calcium channel antagonists. Lung transplantation is reserved for late stages of the disease when patients are unresponsive to prostacyclin. The disease does not appear to recur after transplantation.

144. The answer is d. (*Braunwald, 15/e, pp 1521–1523.*) With the history of daytime sleepiness and snoring at night, the patient requires evaluation for obstructive sleep apnea syndrome. Frequent awakenings are actually more suggestive of central sleep apnea. Polysomnography is required to assess which type of sleep apnea syndrome is present. EEG variables are recorded that identify various stages of sleep. Arterial oxygen saturation is monitored by finger or ear oximetry. Heart rate is monitored. The respiratory pattern is monitored to detect apnea and whether it is central or obstructive. Ambulatory sleep monitoring with oxygen saturation studies alone might identify multiple episodes of desaturation, but negative results would not rule out a sleep apnea syndrome. Overnight oximetry alone can be used in some patients when the index of suspicion for obstructive sleep apnea is high.

145. The answer is a. (*Braunwald, 15/e, pp 1522–1523.*) In this patient with multiple episodes of desaturation, continuous positive airway pressure would be the recommended therapy. Weight loss is often helpful and should be recommended as well, but would probably not be sufficient. Uvulopalatopharyngoplasty has also been used in obstructive sleep apnea, but when applied to unselected patients is effective in less than 50%. Tracheostomy is a course of last resort that does provide immediate relief.

Cardiology

Questions

DIRECTIONS: Each item below contains a question or incomplete statement followed by suggested responses. Select the **one best** response to each question.

146. A 60-year-old male patient on aspirin, nitrates, and a beta blocker, being followed for chronic stable angina, presents to the ER with a history of two to three episodes of more severe and long-lasting anginal chest pain each day over the past 3 days. His ECG and cardiac enzymes are normal. The best course of action of the following is to

a. Admit the patient and begin intravenous digoxin
b. Admit the patient and begin intravenous heparin
c. Admit the patient and give prophylactic thrombolytic therapy
d. Admit the patient for observation with no change in medication
e. Discharge the patient from the ER with increases in nitrates and beta blockers

147. A 60-year-old white female presents with epigastric pain, nausea and vomiting, heart rate of 50, and pronounced first-degree AV block on ER cardiac monitor. Blood pressure is 130/80. The coronary artery most likely to be involved in this process is the

a. Right coronary
b. Left main
c. Left anterior descending
d. Circumflex

148. You are seeing in your office a patient with the chief complaint of relatively sudden onset of shortness of breath and weakness but no chest pain. ECG shows nonspecific ST-T changes. You would be particularly attuned to the possibility of painless, or silent, myocardial infarction in the

a. Advanced coronary artery disease patient with unstable angina on multiple medications
b. Elderly diabetic
c. Premenopausal female
d. Inferior MI patient
e. MI patient with PVCs

149. A 75-year-old African American female is admitted with acute myocardial infarction and congestive heart failure, then has an episode of ventricular tachycardia. She is prescribed multiple medications and soon develops confusion and slurred speech. The most likely cause of this confusion is

a. Captopril
b. Digoxin
c. Furosemide
d. Lidocaine
e. Nitroglycerin

150. Two weeks after hospital discharge for documented myocardial infarction, a 65-year-old returns to your office very concerned about low-grade fever and pleuritic chest pain. There is no associated shortness of breath. Lungs are clear to auscultation and heart exam is free of significant murmurs, gallops, or rubs. ECG is unchanged from the last one in the hospital. The most effective therapy is likely

a. Antibiotics
b. Anticoagulation with warfarin (Coumadin)
c. An anti-inflammatory agent
d. An increase in antianginal medication
e. An antianxiety agent

151. A 72-year-old male presents to the ER with the chief complaint of shortness of breath that awakens him at night and also night cough. Further questioning confirms recent dyspnea on exertion. As you pursue the diagnosis of congestive heart failure using the Framingham criteria, you note the physical exam findings below. Which of the findings is considered among the less specific minor criteria?

a. Neck vein distention
b. Rales
c. S_3 gallop
d. Positive hepatojugular reflux
e. Extremity edema

152. A 55-year-old patient presents to you with a history of having recently had a myocardial infarction with a 5-day hospital stay while away on a business trip. He reports being told he had mild congestive heart failure then, but is asymptomatic now with normal physical exam. You recommend which of the following medications?

a. An ACE inhibitor
b. Digoxin
c. Diltiazem
d. Furosemide (Lasix)
e. Hydralazine plus nitrates

153. A 26-year-old female is referred to you from an OB-GYN colleague due to the onset of extreme fatigue and dyspnea on exertion 3 months after her second vaginal delivery. By history, physical, and echocardiogram, which shows systolic dysfunction, you make the diagnosis of postpartum cardiomyopathy. Which of the following is correct?

a. Postpartum cardiomyopathy may occur unexpectedly years after pregnancy and delivery
b. About half of all patients will recover completely
c. Since the condition is idiosyncratic, future pregnancy may be entered into with no greater than average risk
d. The postpartum state will require a different therapeutic approach than typical dilated cardiomyopathies

154. Yesterday you admitted a 55-year-old white male to the hospital due to chest pain and ruled out MI. The patient tends to be anxious about his health. On admission, his lungs were clear, and his heart revealed a grade II/VI systolic crescendo-decrescendo murmur at the upper right sternal border; cardiac enzymes were normal, and resting ECG showed right bundle branch block with less than 1 mm ST segment depression. The idea of performing a routine Bruce protocol treadmill exercise test (stress test) to further assess coronary artery disease was considered, but rejected primarily due to which of the following?

a. Anticipated difficulty with the patient's anxiety (i.e., he might falsely claim chest pain during the test)
b. Pulmonary embolus suspected as the primary diagnosis
c. Concern about the presence of aortic stenosis, a contraindication to stress testing
d. The presence of RBBB, with this baseline ECG change obscuring typical diagnostic ST-T changes
e. Concern that this represents the onset of unstable angina with unacceptable risk of MI with stress testing

155. A 75-year-old patient presents to the ER after a sudden syncopal episode. He is again alert and in retrospect describes occasional substernal chest pressure and shortness of breath on exertion. His lungs have a few bibasilar rales, and his blood pressure is 110/80. On cardiac auscultation, the classic finding you expect to hear is

a. A harsh systolic crescendo-decrescendo murmur heard best at the upper right sternal border
b. A diastolic decrescendo murmur heard at the mid-left sternal border
c. A holosystolic murmur heard best at the apex
d. A midsystolic click

156. A 72-year-old male comes to the office with intermittent symptoms of dyspnea on exertion, palpitations, and cough occasionally productive of blood. On cardiac auscultation, a low-pitched diastolic rumbling murmur is faintly heard toward the apex. The origin of the patient's problem probably relates to

a. Rheumatic fever as a youth
b. Long-standing hypertension
c. Silent MI within the past year
d. Congenital origin

157. You are helping with school sports physicals and see a 13-year-old boy who has had some trouble keeping up with his peers. He has a cardiac murmur, which you correctly diagnose as a ventricular septal defect based on which of the following auscultatory findings?

a. A systolic crescendo-decrescendo murmur heard best at the upper right sternal border with radiation to the carotids; the murmur is augmented with transient exercise
b. A systolic murmur at the pulmonic area and a diastolic rumble along the left sternal border
c. A holosystolic murmur at the mid-left sternal border
d. A diastolic decrescendo murmur at the mid-left sternal border
e. A continuous murmur through systole and diastole at the upper left sternal border

Items 158–159

158. A 40-year-old male presents to the office with a history of palpitations that last for a few seconds and occur two or three times a week. There are no other symptoms. ECG shows a rare single unifocal premature ventricular contraction (PVC). The most likely cause of this finding is

a. Underlying coronary artery disease
b. Valvular heart disease
c. Hypertension
d. Apathetic hyperthyroidism
e. Idiopathic or unknown

159. Subsequent 24-h Holter monitoring in the preceding patient confirms occasional single unifocal PVCs plus occasional premature atrial contractions (PACs). The best antiarrhythmic management in this case is

a. Anxiolytics
b. Beta blocker therapy
c. Digoxin
d. Quinidine
e. Observation, no medication

160. An active 78-year-old female has been followed for hypertension but presents with new onset of mild left hemiparesis and the finding of atrial fibrillation on ECG, which persists throughout the hospital stay. She had been in sinus rhythm 6 months earlier. Optimal treatment by the time of hospital discharge includes antihypertensives plus

a. Close observation
b. Permanent pacemaker
c. Aspirin
d. Warfarin (Coumadin)
e. Subcutaneous heparin

Items 161–162

161. A 36-year-old white female nurse comes to the ER due to a sensation of fast heart rate, slight dizziness, and vague chest fullness. Blood pressure is 110/70. The following rhythm strip is obtained, which shows

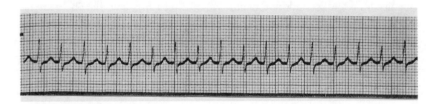

a. Atrial fibrillation
b. Atrial flutter
c. Supraventricular tachycardia
d. Ventricular tachycardia

162. The initial pharmacologic therapy of choice in this stable patient is

a. Adenosine 6 mg rapid IV bolus
b. Verapamil 2.5 to 5 mg IV over 1 to 2 min
c. Diltiazem 0.25 mg/kg IV over 2 min
d. Digoxin 0.5 mg IV slowly
e. Lidocaine 1.5 mg/kg IV bolus
f. Electrical cardioversion at 50 joules

163. A 65-year-old man with diabetes, on an oral hypoglycemic, presents to the ER with a sports-related right shoulder injury. His heart rate was noted to be irregular and the following ECG was obtained. The best immediate therapy is

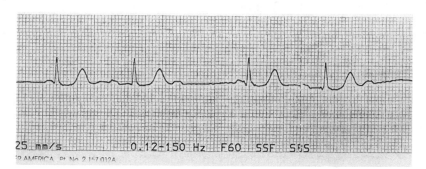

a. Atropine
b. Isoproterenol
c. Pacemaker
d. Electrical cardioversion
e. Digoxin
f. Diltiazem
g. Observation

164. While at the grocery store, you see an elderly lady slump to the floor. Going to her aid, your first step in Adult Basic Life Support (CPR) should be the following

a. Check for a carotid pulse
b. Assess breathing
c. Establish an airway
d. Determine responsiveness
e. Institute chest compression

165. In the ICU, a patient suddenly becomes unresponsive, pulseless, and hypotensive, with cardiac monitor indicating ventricular tachycardia. The crash cart is immediately available. The first therapeutic step among the following should be

a. Amiodarone 300 mg IV push
b. Lidocaine 1.5 mg/kg IV push
c. Epinephrine 1 mg IV push
d. Defibrillation at 200 joules
e. Defibrillation at 360 joules

166. A 55-year-old African American female presents to the ER with lethargy and blood pressure of 250/150. Her family members indicate that she was complaining of severe headache and visual disturbance earlier in the day. They report a past history of asthma but no known kidney disease. On physical exam, papilledema and retinal hemorrhages are present. The best approach is

a. Intravenous labetalol therapy
b. Continuous-infusion nitroprusside
c. Clonidine by mouth to lower blood pressure slowly but surely
d. Nifedipine sublingually to lower blood pressure rapidly and remove the patient from danger
e. Further history about recent home antihypertensives before deciding current therapy

Items 167–168

An 18-year-old male complains of fever and transient pain in both knees and elbows. The right knee was red and swollen for 1 day the week prior to presentation. On physical exam, the patient has a low-grade fever but appears generally well. There is an aortic diastolic murmur heard at the base of the heart. A nodule is palpated over the extensor tendon of the hand. There are pink erythematous lesions over the abdomen, some with central clearing. The following laboratory values are obtained:

Hct: 42
WBC: 12,000/μL
20% polymorphonuclear leukocytes
80% lymphocytes
ESR: 60 mm/h
     The patient's ECG is shown on the facing page.

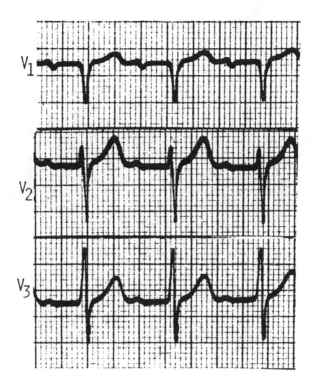

167. Which of the following tests is most critical to diagnosis?

a. Blood cultures
b. Antistreptolysin O antibody
c. Echocardiogram
d. Antinuclear antibodies
e. Creatinine phosphokinase

168. Based on the data available, the best approach to therapy is

a. Ceftriaxone
b. Corticosteroids plus penicillin
c. Acetaminophen
d. Penicillin plus streptomycin
e. Ketoconazole

169. A patient has been in the cardiac care unit with an acute anterior myocardial infarction. He develops the abnormal rhythm shown below. You should

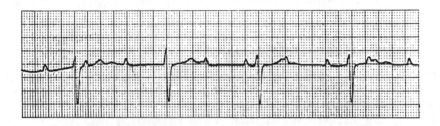

a. Give digoxin
b. Consult for pacemaker
c. Perform cardioversion
d. Give propranolol
e. Give lidocaine

170. A 48-year-old male with a history of hypercholesterolemia presents to the ER after 1 h of substernal chest pain, nausea, and sweating. His ECG is shown at right. There is no history of hypertension, stroke, or any other serious illness. Which of the following therapies is not appropriate?

a. Aspirin
b. Beta blocker
c. Morphine
d. Digoxin
e. Nitroglycerin
f. Thrombolytic agent

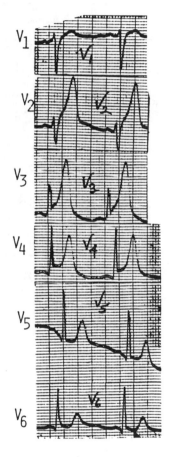

171. A 55-year-old obese woman develops pressurelike substernal chest pain 1 h in duration. Her ECG is shown below. The most likely diagnosis is

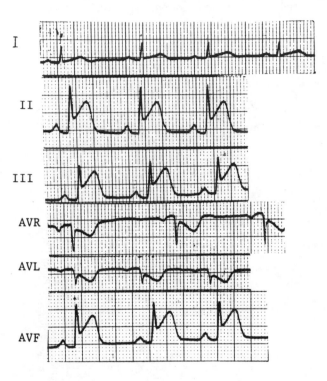

a. Costochondritis
b. Acute anterior myocardial infarction
c. Acute inferior myocardial infarction
d. Pericarditis
e. Esophageal reflux
f. Cholecystitis

172. A 50-year-old construction worker continues to have an elevated blood pressure of 160/95 even after a third agent is added to his antihypertensive regimen. Physical exam is normal, electrolytes are normal, and the patient is taking no over-the-counter medications. The next helpful step for this patient is to

a. Check pill count
b. Evaluate for Cushing syndrome
c. Check chest x-ray for coarctation of the aorta
d. Obtain a renal angiogram
e. Obtain an adrenal CT scan

Items 173–174

A 35-year-old male complains of substernal chest pain aggravated by inspiration and relieved by sitting up. He has a history of tuberculosis. Lung fields are clear to auscultation, and heart sounds are somewhat distant. Chest x-ray shows an enlarged cardiac silhouette.

173. The next step in evaluation is

a. Right lateral decubitus film
b. Cardiac catheterization
c. Echocardiogram
d. Serial ECGs
e. Thallium stress test

174. The patient then develops jugular venous distention and hypotension. The ECG shows electrical alternans. The most likely additional physical finding is

a. Basilar rales halfway up both posterior lung fields
b. S_3 gallop
c. Pulsus paradoxus
d. Strong apical beat

175. A 43-year-old woman with a 1-year history of episodic leg edema and dyspnea is noted to have clubbing of the fingers. Her ECG is shown below. The correct diagnosis is

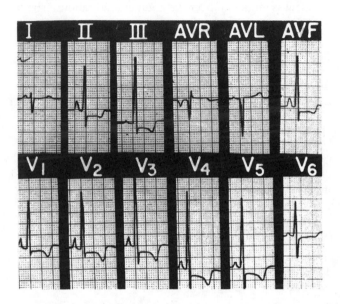

a. Inferior wall myocardial infarction
b. Right bundle branch block
c. Acute pericarditis
d. Wolff-Parkinson-White syndrome
e. Cor pulmonale

176. A 62-year-old male with underlying COPD develops a viral upper respiratory infection and begins taking an over-the-counter decongestant. Shortly thereafter he experiences palpitations and presents to the emergency room, where the following rhythm strip is obtained, demonstrating

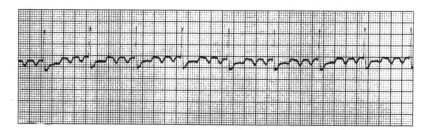

a. Normal sinus rhythm
b. Junctional rhythm
c. Atrial flutter with 4:1 atrioventricular block
d. Paroxysmal atrial tachycardia with 2:1 atrioventricular block
e. Complete heart block with 2:1 atrioventricular block

177. An asymptomatic 30-year-old female was noted by her gynecologist to have a cardiac murmur. She was referred for an echocardiogram, with results reported to her as showing mitral valve prolapse. The patient desires more information and now comes to you. Which of the following is true about her condition?

a. Echocardiography demonstrates displacement of one or both mitral valve leaflets posteriorly into the left atrium during systole
b. Migration of the systolic click and systolic murmur toward the first heart sound will occur during squatting
c. Prophylactic beta blocker therapy is indicated
d. Significant mitral regurgitation is likely to occur (>50% chance) sometime in her life
e. Restriction of exercise is advised to reduce the risk of sudden cardiac death

178. You are reviewing a number of patients with congenital heart disease with specific attention to whether or not they need antibiotic prophylaxis for dental work. Which of the following cardiac conditions creates the lowest risk for development of infective endocarditis?

a. Coarctation of the aorta
b. Ventricular septal defect
c. Atrial septal defect
d. Patent ductus arteriosus
e. Prosthetic heart valve

179. An 80-year-old with a past history of myocardial infarction is found to have left bundle branch block on ECG. He is asymptomatic with blood pressure 130/80, lungs clear to auscultation, and no leg edema. On cardiac auscultation, the most likely finding is

a. Fixed (wide) split S_2
b. Paradoxical (reversed) split S_2
c. S_3
d. S_4
e. Opening snap
f. Midsystolic click

DIRECTIONS: Each group of questions below consists of lettered options followed by a set of numbered items. For each numbered item, select the **one** lettered option with which it is **most** closely associated. Each lettered option may be used once, more than once, or not at all.

Items 180–182

You are assisting for 1 month in a cardiology valvular heart disease clinic, detecting a variety of murmurs and associated features. Match the physical findings with the most likely valvular or related heart disease.

a. Mitral stenosis
b. Tricuspid regurgitation
c. Mitral regurgitation
d. Aortic regurgitation
e. Aortic stenosis
f. Hypertrophic cardiomyopathy

180. High-pitched, blowing, decrescendo diastolic murmur; widened arterial pulse pressure **(SELECT 1 DISORDER)**

181. Holosystolic murmur at left sternal border; increased murmur on inspiration; prominent V wave in neck **(SELECT 1 DISORDER)**

182. Crescendo-decrescendo systolic murmur beginning well after S_1, heard best at the lower left sternal border; rapidly rising carotid arterial pulse **(SELECT 1 DISORDER)**

Items 183–186

While on call in the hospital, you become involved in the following emergent situations. For each clinical setting, choose the best next step in management from the following choices.

a. Digoxin
b. Propranolol
c. Calcium channel blocker
d. Atropine
e. Heparin
f. Lidocaine
g. Isoproterenol
h. Observation

183. Two-hour history of chest pain; acute ST segment elevation in leads 2, 3, and AVF; sinus bradycardia at rate of 40 with hypotension **(SELECT 1 STEP)**

184. Sudden onset of chest pain at night; ST segment elevations in precordial leads that resolve with sublingual nitroglycerin **(SELECT 1 STEP)**

185. Development of accelerated idioventricular rhythm post–myocardial infarction, with rate of 80 **(SELECT 1 STEP)**

186. Shortness of breath, palpitations, bifid apical beat, and increased intensity of systolic murmur on Valsalva maneuver **(SELECT 1 STEP)**

Items 187–190

In the outpatient setting, you are treating a number of patients with hypertension. Knowing the adverse possibilities along with the benefits of each antihypertensive can help you achieve compliance and therefore blood pressure control. Match the cardiac and/or antihypertensive agents below with their associated side effects.

a. Increased triglyceride levels
b. Volume retention
c. Lupus-like syndrome
d. Cough
e. Gynecomastia
f. Rebound hypertension
g. First-dose syncope
h. Urinary retention

187. Captopril **(SELECT 1 EFFECT)**

188. Propranolol **(SELECT 1 EFFECT)**

189. Spironolactone **(SELECT 1 EFFECT)**

190. Terazosin **(SELECT 1 EFFECT)**

Items 191–194

You have been assigned to review the ECGs for the group this month. Many of the patients have renal problems and/or hypertension. For each electrolyte abnormality below, select the electrocardiographic finding with which it is most commonly associated.

a. No known electrocardiographic abnormalities
b. Prolonged QT interval
c. Short QT interval
d. Widened QRS complex
e. Prominent U waves

191. Hypokalemia **(SELECT 1 ECG FINDING)**

192. Hyperkalemia **(SELECT 1 ECG FINDING)**

193. Hypocalcemia **(SELECT 1 ECG FINDING)**

194. Hyponatremia **(SELECT 1 ECG FINDING)**

Cardiology

Answers

146. The answer is b. *(Fuster, 10/e, pp 1246–1264.)* This patient presents with unstable angina, a change from the previous chronic stable state in that chest pain has become more frequent and more severe. Intravenous heparin is indicated. Subcutaneous administration of low-molecular-weight heparin (such as enoxaparin) is an alternative. There is no role for digoxin, as this may increase myocardial oxygen consumption and exacerbate the situation. Thrombolytic therapy is reserved for the treatment, typically within 6 h, of ECG-documented myocardial infarction and does not reduce cardiac events in the setting of unstable angina. A more aggressive approach is early interventional cardiac catheterization with angioplasty and/or stent placement, possibly in conjunction with glycoprotein IIb/IIIa inhibitors.

147. The answer is a. *(Fuster, 10/e, pp 52, 88.)* The right coronary artery supplies most of the inferior myocardium and supplies the AV node in over 70% of patients. Thus occlusion of this artery can cause ischemia of the AV node with AV block or bradycardia, as well as symptoms of an inferior MI as seen in this patient. AV block can occur with anterior MI related to LAD occlusion, but this generally implies a greater area of myocardial involvement and hemodynamic instability.

148. The answer is b. *(Braunwald, 15/e, p 1387.)* The classic presentation of acute myocardial infarction (MI) involves heavy or crushing substernal chest pain or pressure. However, 15 to 20% of infarctions may be painless, with the greatest incidence in diabetics and the elderly. Dyspnea or weakness may initially predominate in these patients. Other presentations include altered mental status, the appearance of an arrhythmia, or hypotension. Diabetics are likely to have abnormal or absent pain response to myocardial ischemia due to generalized autonomic nervous system dysfunction. The other choices have no specific link to greater likelihood of a silent MI.

149. The answer is d. *(Fuster, 10/e, pp 902–905.)* While the clinical picture itself could lead to these neurological symptoms, the only cardiovascular medication on this list likely to do so is lidocaine. Lidocaine is particularly likely to cause confusion in the elderly patient, for whom a lower dose of the drug should generally be given. Other potential adverse effects of lidocaine include tremor, convulsions, respiratory depression, bradycardia, and hypotension.

150. The answer is c. (*Braunwald, 15/e, p 1369.*) The history and physical are consistent with post–cardiac injury syndrome (in the past also known as Dressler syndrome or postmyocardial infarction syndrome). This generally benign self-limited syndrome comprises an autoimmune pleuritis, pneumonitis, or pericarditis characterized by fever and pleuritic chest pain, with onset days to 6 weeks post cardiac injury with blood in the pericardial cavity, as after a cardiac operation, cardiac trauma, or MI. Therefore the most effective therapy is a nonsteroidal anti-inflammatory drug or occasionally a glucocorticoid. Infection such as bacterial pneumonia, which would require antibiotics, would typically cause dyspnea, cough with sputum production, and rales on lung auscultation. Pulmonary embolus, which would require anticoagulation, would cause dyspnea and tachypnea, often in conjunction with physical findings of heat, swelling, and pain in the leg consistent with deep vein thrombosis. Angina or recurrent myocardial infarction is always a concern post MI (and what the patient usually fears in this situation), but the nature of the pain—here pleuritic rather than pressurelike—and the unchanged ECG are fairly reassuring and mitigate against an increase in antianginal therapy. Anxiety can be present but would not cause fever.

151. The answer is e. (*Braunwald, 15/e, pp 1322–1323.*) Use of the Framingham criteria (eight major and seven minor) is one method by which to organize the signs and symptoms for the diagnosis of congestive heart failure. Major criteria include paroxysmal nocturnal dyspnea, neck vein distension, rales, cardiomegaly, acute pulmonary edema, S_3 gallop, increased venous pressure, and hepatojugular reflux. Minor criteria include extremity edema, night cough, dyspnea on exertion, hepatomegaly, pleural effusion, vital capacity reduced by one-third from normal, and tachycardia of 120 or more beats per minute. In addition, weight loss of 4.5 kg or more over 5 days of treatment may be considered as a major or minor criterion. To establish a clinical diagnosis of congestive heart failure, at least one major and two minor criteria are required.

152. The answer is a. (*Braunwald, 15/e, pp 1323–1327.*) The administration of an angiotensin converting enzyme inhibitor has been shown to prevent or retard the development of heart failure in patients with left ventricular dysfunction and to reduce long-term mortality when begun shortly after an MI. This relates to inhibition of the renin-angiotensin system and to reduction of preload and afterload. Other agents that might be considered for prevention of deterioration of myocardial function include a beta blocker, an angiotensin II receptor blocker, and/or an aldosterone antagonist such as spironolactone. General therapeutic measures also include salt restriction and regular moderate exercise. Digoxin is reserved for those with clear-cut systolic dysfunction. Calcium channel blockers are not indicated for heart failure or routinely post MI. Loop or thiazide diuretics are administered in those with fluid accumulation. The nitrate-hydralazine combination is an option in ACE inhibitor–intolerant patients.

153. The answer is b. (*Fuster, 10/e, p 1958.*) Postpartum (or peripartum) cardiomyopathy may occur during the last trimester of pregnancy or within 6 months of delivery. About half of patients will recover completely, with most of the rest improving. However, current advice is to avoid future pregnancies due to risk of recurrence. Treatment is as for other dilated cardiomyopathies, except that ACE inhibitors are contraindicated in pregnancy.

154. The answer is c. (*Fuster, 10/e, pp 469–470, 475–476.*) Cardiac auscultation suggests aortic stenosis, a contraindication to stress testing. This could be evaluated further with echocardiography. Anxiety or suspected angina would not preclude a stress test. Pulmonary embolus is not likely by history and physical. ST segment depression is the most common stress test–induced manifestation of myocardial ischemia. This type of change is difficult to assess in the presence of any bundle branch block in which the ST segment is already abnormal. However, updated American College of Cardiology/American Heart Association guidelines do support the use of exercise stress testing in RBBB if the ST segment depression is 1 mm or less. Radionuclide imaging would need to be considered to assess for angina in the setting of LBBB, WPW, paced rhythm, or RBBB with >1 mm resting ST segment depression.

155. The answer is a. (*Braunwald, 15/e, pp 1349–1350.*) The classic symptoms of aortic stenosis are exertional dyspnea, angina pectoris, and syncope. Physical findings include a narrow pulse pressure and systolic murmur as described in option a (rather than the aortic insufficiency murmur of option b, the mitral regurgitation murmur of option c, or the mitral valve prolapse click of option d).

156. The answer is a. *(Braunwald, 15/e, pp 1343–1345.)* The history and physical exam findings are consistent with mitral stenosis. Dyspnea may be present secondary to pulmonary edema; palpitations are often related to atrial arrhythmias (PACs, PAT, atrial flutter or fibrillation); hemoptysis may occur as a consequence of pulmonary hypertension with rupture of bronchial veins. A diastolic rumbling apical murmur is characteristic. An accentuated first heart sound and opening snap may also be present. The etiology of mitral stenosis is usually rheumatic, rarely congenital. Two-thirds of patients afflicted are women.

157. The answer is c. *(Braunwald, 15/e, pp 207–211, 1260–1261, 1335–1336.)* A holosystolic murmur at the mid-left sternal border is the murmur most characteristic of a ventricular septal defect. Both the murmur of ventricular septal defect and the murmur of mitral regurgitation are enhanced by exercise and diminished by amyl nitrite. Options a, b, d, and e describe the usual findings in aortic stenosis, atrial septal defect, aortic insufficiency, and patent ductus arteriosus, respectively.

158. The answer is e. *(Braunwald, 15/e, p 1293.)* PVCs are common in patients with and without heart disease, and are detected in 60% of adult males on Holter monitoring. Occasional unifocal PVCs do not suggest any of the underlying diseases described.

159. The answer is e. *(Braunwald, 15/e, p 1294.)* Minimally symptomatic PVCs do not require treatment. Antiarrhythmic therapy in this setting has not been shown to reduce sudden cardiac death or overall mortality. A beta blocker would be the best choice if symptoms began to interfere with daily activities.

160. The answer is d. *(Braunwald, 15/e, p 1296.)* Aspirin alone might be sufficient for a stroke patient without the complicating factor of atrial fibrillation. However, in patients with atrial fibrillation, in whom the risk of stroke approaches 30%, therapeutic anticoagulation with warfarin (Coumadin) reduces the incidence of future stroke to a greater extent than the use of aspirin. This particular patient may be a candidate for medical or electrical cardioversion, which requires pretreatment with Coumadin for 3 weeks (if the atrial fibrillation has been present for over 48 h or is of unknown onset). Alternatively, a transesophageal echocardiogram (TEE) could be performed to exclude the presence of left atrial thrombus, followed by cardioversion and then maintenance warfarin anticoagulation for 4 weeks.

161. The answer is c. *(Fuster, 10/e, pp 809–812, 820–825, 837–841.)* Paroxysmal supraventricular tachycardia due to AV nodal reentry typically displays a narrow QRS complex without clearly discernable P waves, with a rate in the 160 to 190 range. The atrial rate is faster in atrial flutter, typically with a classic sawtooth pattern of P waves, with AV conduction ratios most commonly 2:1 or 4:1, leading to ventricular rates of 150 or 75/min. Atrial fibrillation would show an irregularly irregular rhythm. Wide QRS complexes would be expected in ventricular tachycardia.

162. The answer is a. *(Fuster, 10/e, pp 812–815.)* Vagotonic maneuvers such as carotid massage or the Valsalva maneuver could certainly be tried first. If these are unsuccessful, adenosine, with its excellent safety profile and extremely short half-life, is the drug of choice for supraventricular tachycardia at an initial dose of 6 mg. Dosage can be repeated if necessary a few minutes later at 12 mg. Verapamil is the next alternative; if the initial dose of 2.5 to 5 mg does not yield conversion, one or two additional boluses 10 min apart can be used. Diltiazem and digoxin may be useful in rate control and conversion, but have a much slower onset of action. Electrical cardioversion would be reserved for hemodynamically unstable patients. Lidocaine is useful in ventricular, not supraventricular, arrhythmias.

163. The answer is g. *(Braunwald, 15/e, p 1287.)* This ECG shows Mobitz type I second-degree AV block, also known as Wenckebach phenomenon, characterized by progressive PR interval prolongation prior to block of an atrial impulse. This rhythm generally does not require therapy. It may be seen in normal individuals; other causes include inferior MI and drug intoxications such as from digoxin, beta blockers, or calcium channel blockers. Even in the post-MI setting, it is usually stable, although it has the potential to progress to higher-degree AV block with consequent need for pacemaker.

164. The answer is d. (*Cummins, 1/e, pp 5–6.*) One cannot automatically assume initially that an individual has had a cardiac or respiratory arrest. Therefore, first determine responsiveness by tapping or gently shaking the victim and shouting, "Are you OK?" Then proceed with the ACLS approach. Shout or phone for help, then position the victim and yourself. Follow this with the **ABCDs** (establishing the **A**irway, assessing **B**reathing, assessing **C**irculation, and managing any need for **D**efibrillation).

165. The answer is d. (*Cummins, 1/e, pp 77–78, 82–83.*) The standard approach to ventricular fibrillation or pulseless ventricular tachycardia involves defibrillation with 200 joules, then 300, then 360, followed if needed by epinephrine 1 mg IV push every 3 to 5 min. Persistent ventricular fibrillation or pulseless ventricular tachycardia leads to consideration of amiodarone 300 mg IV push or lidocaine 1.0 to 1.5 mg/kg IV push. In addition, magnesium sulfate 1 to 2 g IV may be given in torsade de pointes or when arrhythmia due to hypomagnesemia is suspected. Procainamide up to 50 mg/min (maximum total 17 mg/kg) is given to patients with intermittent return of a pulse or non-VF rhythm, but then recurrence of VF/VT. A precordial thump may be considered in this setting, but there is insufficient evidence to recommend its use or avoidance.

166. The answer is b. (*Braunwald, 15/e, p 1428–1429.*) This patient manifests malignant hypertension with diastolic blood pressure >130 and acute (or ongoing) target organ damage. She shows one subset of such damage, namely hypertensive encephalopathy, including headache, visual disturbance, and altered mental status. Immediate therapy with nitroprusside is indicated in the ICU setting, although it would be avoided if renal insufficiency were present. Other options include intravenous nitroglycerin or intravenous enalaprilat. Intravenous labetalol is often used in hypertensive urgencies, but, as a beta blocker, it is relatively contraindicated in asthma. An oral medication such as clonidine would be difficult and slow-acting in a lethargic patient. Sublingual nifedipine is no longer advised due to increased potential for overshoot hypotension with adverse cardiovascular events such as MI or stroke, and ischemic optic neuropathy.

167–168. The answers are 167-b, 168-b. (*Braunwald, 15/e, pp 1340–1342.*) This 18-year-old presents with classic features of rheumatic fever. His clinical manifestations include arthritis, fever, and murmur. A subcutaneous nodule is noted, and a rash of erythema marginatum is described. These subcutaneous nodules are pea-sized and usually seen over extensor tendons. The rash is usually pink with clear centers and serpiginous margins. Laboratory data shows an elevated erythrocyte sedimentation rate as usually occurs in rheumatic fever. The ECG shows evidence of first-degree AV block. An antistreptolysin O antibody is necessary to diagnose the disease by documenting prior streptococcal infection. Most experts recommend the use of glucocorticoids when carditis is part of the picture of rheumatic fever. Therefore, in this patient with first-degree AV block, corticosteroids would be indicated. Penicillin should also be given to eradicate group A β-hemolytic streptococci.

169. The answer is b. (*Braunwald, 15/e, pp 1287–1290.*) The ECG shows complete heart block. Although at first glance the P waves and QRS complexes may appear related, on closer inspection they are completely independent of each other, i.e., dissociated. Complete heart block in the setting of acute myocardial infarction requires at least temporary, and often permanent, transvenous pacemaker placement. Atropine may be used as a temporary measure. You would certainly want to avoid digoxin, beta blockers, or any other medication that promotes bradycardia. There is no indication on this strip for cardioversion such as for atrial fibrillation/flutter or ventricular tachycardia/fibrillation. Lidocaine would be relatively contraindicated in that it might suppress the ventricular pacemaker, leading to asystole.

170. The answer is d. (*Braunwald, 15/e, pp 1389–1392.*) The ECG shows acute ST segment elevations in the anterior precordial leads. The symptoms have persisted for only 1 h and the patient does not seem to have any contraindications to thrombolytic therapy, which may be given along with aspirin. Nitroglycerin and morphine are indicated for pain control. Beta blockers reduce pain, limit infarct size, and decrease ventricular arrhythmias. There is no role for digoxin in this acute setting; in fact, it may increase myocardial oxygen consumption and increase infarct size.

171. The answer is c. (*Braunwald, 15/e, pp 1267–1269.*) The ECG shows ST segment elevation in inferior leads II, III, and a VF with reciprocal ST depression in a VL, which is highly consistent with an acute inferior MI. An anterior MI would produce ST segment elevation in the precordial leads. Pericarditis classically produces pleuritic chest pain and diffuse ST segment elevation (except aVR) on ECG. Costochondritis, esophageal reflux, cholecystitis, and duodenal ulcer disease can all cause the symptoms of substernal chest pain, but not these ECG findings.

172. The answer is a. *(Braunwald, 15/e, p 1428.)* The most common cause of refractory hypertension is nonadherence to the medication regimen. A history from the patient is useful, and pill count is the best compliance check. Cushing's disease, coarctation of the aorta, renal artery stenosis, and primary aldosteronism are secondary causes that could result in refractory hypertension, but no clues to these diagnoses are apparent on physical exam or lab.

173. The answer is c. *(Braunwald, 15/e, pp 1365–1366.)* The patient's pleuritic chest pain that is relieved by sitting up is most likely due to pericarditis. A pericardial friction rub may initially be present, then disappear, with the heart sounds becoming fainter as an effusion develops. Lung sounds are typically clear. An enlarged cardiac silhouette without other chest x-ray findings of heart failure suggests pericardial effusion.

Echocardiography is the most sensitive, specific way of determining whether pericardial fluid is present. The effusion appears as an echo-free space between the moving epicardium and stationary pericardium. It is unnecessary to perform cardiac catheterization for the purpose of evaluating pericardial effusion. Radionuclide scanning is not a preferred method for demonstrating pericardial fluid.

174. The answer is c. *(Braunwald, 15/e, pp 1367–1368.)* The patient has developed cardiac tamponade, a condition in which pericardial fluid under increased pressure impedes diastolic filling, resulting in reduced cardiac output and hypotension. On exam there is elevation of jugular venous pressure. The jugular venous pulse shows a sharp x descent, the inward impulse seen at the time of the carotid pulsation. An important confirmatory clue to cardiac tamponade on exam is pulsus paradoxus, a greater than normal (10 mmHg) inspiratory decline in systolic arterial pressure. In contrast to pulmonary edema, the lungs are usually clear. Neither a strong apical beat nor an S_3 gallop would be expected in tamponade.

175. The answer is e. *(Fuster, 10/e, pp 1616–1619.)* Cor pulmonale is characterized by the presence of pulmonary hypertension and consequent right ventricular dysfunction. Its causes include diseases leading to hypoxic vasoconstriction, as in cystic fibrosis; occlusion of the pulmonary vasculature, as in pulmonary thromboembolism; and parenchymal destruction, as in sarcoidosis. In the presence of a chronic increase in afterload, the right ventricle becomes hypertrophic, dilates, and fails. The electrocardiographic findings, as illustrated in the question, include tall, peaked P waves in leads II, III, and a VF, which indicate right atrial enlargement; tall R waves in leads V_1 to V_3 and a deep S wave in V_6 with associated ST-T wave changes, which indicate right ventricular hypertrophy; and right axis deviation. Right bundle branch block occurs in 15% of patients.

176. The answer is c. *(Braunwald, 15/e, p 1297.)* The rhythm strip in the question reveals atrial flutter with 4:1 atrioventricular (AV) block. Atrial flutter is characterized by an atrial rate of 250 to 350/min; the electrocardiogram typically reveals a sawtooth baseline configuration due to the flutter waves. In the strip, every fourth atrial depolarization is conducted through the AV node, resulting in a ventricular rate of 75/min (although 2:1 conduction is more commonly seen).

177. The answer is a. *(Braunwald, 15/e, pp 1348–1349.)* The fundamental defect in mitral valve prolapse is an abnormality of the valve's connective tissue with secondary proliferation of myxomatous tissue. The redundant leaflet(s) prolapses toward the left atrium in systole, which results in the auscultated click and murmur and characteristic echocardiographic findings. Any maneuver that reduces left ventricular size, such as standing or the Valsalva maneuver, allows the click and murmur to occur earlier in systole; conversely, conditions that increase left ventricular size, such as squatting or propranolol administration, delay the onset of the click and murmur. Severe mitral regurgitation is an uncommon complication. Most patients with MVP have a benign prognosis, and, in the absence of mitral regurgitation or arrhythmias, reassurance is the key point in management. Antibiotic prophylaxis to prevent endocarditis is reserved for those with the systolic murmur of mitral regurgitation and/or thickening of mitral valve leaflets on echocardiography. Beta blocker therapy is reserved for symptoms, including those related to arrhythmias.

178. The answer is c. (*Fuster, 10/e, p 2089.*) The list of conditions carrying a relatively high risk for development of infective endocarditis includes Marfan syndrome, prosthetic heart valves, coarctation of the aorta, aortic valve disease, ventricular septal defect, mitral insufficiency, and patent ductus arteriosus. Mitral valve prolapse, pure mitral stenosis, and tricuspid and pulmonic valve disease are among the conditions conferring intermediate risk. Among the conditions considered to entail very low risk are atrial septal defect, syphilitic aortitis, and cardiac pacemakers.

179. The answer is b. (*Braunwald, 15/e, pp 1258–1259.*) Normally, the second heart sound (S_2) is composed of aortic closure followed by pulmonic closure. Because inspiration increases blood return to the right side of the heart, pulmonic closure is delayed, which results in normal splitting of S_2 during inspiration. Paradoxical splitting of S_2, however, refers to splitting of S_2 that is narrowed instead of widened with inspiration consequent to a delayed aortic closure. Paradoxical splitting can result from any electrical or mechanical event that delays left ventricular systole. Thus, aortic stenosis and hypertension, which increase resistance to systolic ejection of blood, delay closure of the aortic valve. Acute ischemia from angina or acute myocardial infarction also can delay ejection of blood from the left ventricle. The most common cause of paradoxical splitting—left bundle branch block—delays electrical activation of the left ventricle. Right bundle branch block results in a wide splitting of S_2 that widens further during inspiration. An S_3 is typically heard with congestive heart failure, an S_4 with hypertension, an opening snap with mitral stenosis, and a midsystolic click with mitral valve prolapse.

180–182. The answers are 180-d, 181-b, 182-f. (*Braunwald, 15/e, pp 1260–1261, 1352–1354, 1362.*) The diastolic murmur described is characteristic of aortic regurgitation. Unless it is very minor in magnitude, the aortic regurgitant murmur will be accompanied by peripheral signs such as widened pulse pressure. A holosystolic murmur that is increased on inspiration is the result of tricuspid insufficiency. The neck veins are usually distended with prominent V waves and signs of right-sided heart failure. The final description is of hypertrophic cardiomyopathy, which may also be heard at the apex, where it is more holosystolic. These patients have diffuse left ventricular hypertrophy with preferential hypertrophy of the interventricular septum and a dynamic LV outflow tract pressure gradient.

183–186. The answers are 183-d, 184-c, 185-h, 186-b. *(Braunwald, 15/e, pp 1362–1363, 1397, 1408.)* Sinus bradycardia is a common rhythm disturbance in acute inferior MI, secondary to vagal tone. With associated hypotension, atropine should be given. Intravenous inotropic agents are generally not required. The syndrome of sudden onset of chest pain at night in association with ST segment elevation was initially described by Prinzmetal. Classically, the syndrome is caused by coronary artery spasm, often in smokers and in a younger age group than typical angina patients. Calcium channel blockers are the agents of choice. Accelerated idioventricular rhythm develops in up to 25% of post-MI patients. Enhanced automaticity of Purkinje fibers is considered the most likely etiology. This is usually considered a benign rhythm, and only observation is necessary. The physical findings described in the final clinical scenario strongly suggest the diagnosis of hypertrophic cardiomyopathy. β-adrenergic agents have been used extensively and are considered the agents of choice, especially in the setting of palpitations. Amiodarone is also effective in reducing the incidence of arrhythmias. Among the calcium channel blockers, diltiazem and verapamil (but not nifedipine) may be helpful. Digoxin should be avoided. Hypovolemia as with dehydration or diuretics may also cause deterioration in the hemodynamic status. Strenuous physical activity including competitive sports should generally be limited.

187–190. The answers are 187-d, 188-a, 189-e, 190-g. *(Braunwald, 15/e, pp 1422–1423.)* Captopril which inhibits the angiotensin converting enzyme, is a potent antihypertensive agent because it prevents the generation of angiotensin II, a vasoconstrictor, and inhibits the degradation of bradykinin, a vasodilator. It may cause membranous glomerulopathy, the nephrotic syndrome, and leukopenia. The most common side effect is cough. Propranolol is a nonselective beta blocker and may therefore cause bronchospasm in susceptible patients. Beta blockers, as a class, may reduce HDL cholesterol and increase serum triglyceride levels. Spironolactone, a potassium-sparing diuretic, and methyldopa, a centrally acting antiadrenergic agent, are two antihypertensives that may cause gynecomastia. Alpha blockers such as terazosin may rarely (in <1%) cause first-dose syncope; they may improve, not cause, urinary retention. Volume retention is associated with minoxidil, lupus-like syndrome with hydralazine, and rebound hypertension with clonidine.

191–194. The answers are 191-e, 192-d, 193-b, 194-a. *(Braunwald, 15/e, p 1269.)* Hypokalemia typically increases automaticity of myocardial fibers, which results in ectopic beats or arrhythmias. Electrocardiography in hypokalemia reveals flattening of the T wave and prominent U waves. Hyperkalemia decreases the rate of spontaneous diastolic depolarization in all pacemaker cells. It also results in slowing of conduction. One of the earliest electrocardiographic signs of hyperkalemia is the appearance of tall, peaked T waves. More severe elevations of the serum potassium result in widening of the QRS complex. Hypocalcemia results in prolongation of the QT interval. Low serum calcium levels may also be associated with a decrease in myocardial contractility. At serum sodium levels compatible with life, neither hyponatremia nor hypernatremia results in any characteristic electrocardiographic abnormalities.

Endocrinology and Metabolic Disease

Questions

DIRECTIONS: Each item below contains a question or incomplete statement followed by suggested responses. Select the **one best** response to each question.

Items 195–196

195. A 50-year-old obese female is taking oral hypoglycemic agents. While being treated for an upper respiratory infection, she develops lethargy and is brought to the emergency room. On physical exam, there is no focal neurologic finding or neck rigidity. Laboratory results are as follows:

Na^-: 134 meq/L
K^-: 4.0 meq/L
HCO_3: 25 meq/L
Glucose: 900 mg/dL
BUN: 84 mg/dL
Creatinine: 3.0 mg/dL
BP: 120/80 sitting, 105/65 lying down

The most likely cause of this patient's coma is

a. Diabetic ketoacidosis
b. Hyperosmolar coma
c. Inappropriate ADH
d. Bacterial meningitis

196. The most important treatment in this patient is

a. Large volumes of fluid, insulin; seek concurrent illnesses
b. Bicarbonate infusion 100 meq/L
c. Rapid glucose lowering with intravenous insulin
d. KCL 30 meq/h

197. A 50-year-old female is 5 ft 7 in. tall and weighs 165 lb. There is a family history of diabetes mellitus. Fasting blood glucose is 150 mg/dL on two occasions. She is asymptomatic, and physical exam shows no abnormalities. The treatment of choice is

a. Observation
b. Medical nutrition therapy
c. Insulin
d. Oral hypoglycemic agent

Items 198–200

198. A 30-year-old female complains of palpitations, fatigue, and insomnia. On physical exam, her extremities are warm and she is tachycardic. There is diffuse thyroid gland enlargement and proptosis. There is a thickening of the skin in the pretibial area (see photo). Which of the following lab values would you expect in this patient?

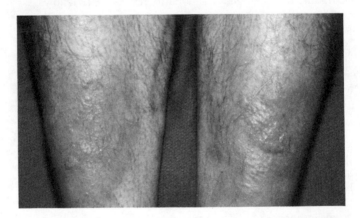

a. Increased TSH, total thyroxine, total T_3
b. Decreased TSH, increased total thyroxine
c. Increased T_3 uptake, decreased T_3
d. Decreased TSH, normal T_4

199. The cause of this patient's thyrotoxicosis is

a. Autoimmune disease
b. Benign tumor
c. Malignancy
d. Viral infection of the thyroid

200. The treatment of choice in this patient, for whom remission from Graves' disease is possible, is

a. Methimazole
b. Radioactive iodine
c. Thyroid surgery
d. Oral corticosteroids

Items 201–203

201. A 30-year-old female complains of fatigue, constipation, and weight gain. There is no prior history of neck surgery or radiation. Her voice is hoarse and her skin is dry. Serum TSH is elevated and T_4 is low. The most likely cause of these findings is

a. Autoimmune disease
b. Postablative hypothyroidism
c. Pituitary hypofunction
d. Thyroid carcinoma

202. Autoimmune thyroiditis can be confirmed in this patient by

a. Thyroid peroxidase antibody (TPO)
b. Antinuclear antibody
c. Thyroid uptake resin
d. Thyroid aspiration

203. On routine physical exam, a young woman is found to have a thyroid nodule. There is no pain, hoarseness, hemoptysis, or local symptoms. Serum TSH is normal. The next step in evaluation is

a. Ultrasonography
b. Thyroid scan
c. Surgical resection
d. Fine needle aspiration of thyroid

DIRECTIONS: Each group of questions below consists of lettered options followed by a set of numbered items. For each numbered item, select the **one** lettered option with which it is **most** closely associated. Each lettered option may be used once, more than once, or not at all.

Items 204–206

Select the most likely disease process for the clinical syndromes described.

a. Acromegaly
b. Prolactin-secreting adenoma
c. Cushing's disease
d. Empty sella syndrome
e. TSH-secreting adenoma
f. Diabetes insipidus

204. A 30-year-old woman has cervical fat pad, purple striae, and hirsutism. **(SELECT 1 DISEASE)**

205. A nonpregnant woman has bitemporal hemianopsia, irregular menses, and galactorrhea. **(SELECT 1 DISEASE)**

206. An obese hypertensive woman has chronic headaches and normal pituitary function. **(SELECT 1 DISEASE)**

207. A 55-year-old type 2 diabetic patient has lost weight and has had good control of his blood sugar on oral agents. He has a history of mild hypertension and hyperlipidemia. He asks for advice about an exercise program. Which one of the following statements is correct?

a. Exercise should be avoided because it may cause foot trauma
b. An active lifestyle cannot slow the complications of diabetes
c. Vigorous exercise cannot precipitate hypoglycemia
d. A stress test should be recommended prior to beginning an exercise program

208. A newly diagnosed type 2 diabetic patient asks for clarification about dietary management. Which of the following is good advice?

a. Restrict carbohydrates and eat a high-protein diet
b. Avoid sucrose altogether
c. Less than 10% of caloric intake should be saturated fat
d. Caloric intake should be very consistent from one day to another

209. As part of a review of systems, a 55-year-old male describes an inability to achieve erection. The patient has mild diabetes and is on a beta blocker for hypertension. The first step in evaluation is

a. Serum testosterone
b. Serum gonadotropin
c. Information about libido and morning erections
d. Papaverine injection

Items 210–212

210. A 90-year-old male complains of hip and back pain. He has also developed headaches, hearing loss, and tinnitus. On physical exam the skull appears enlarged, with prominent superficial veins. There is marked kyphosis, and the bones of the leg appear deformed. Plasma alkaline phosphatase is elevated. A skull x-ray shows sharply demarcated lucencies in the frontal, parietal, and occipital bones. X-rays of the hip show thickening of the pelvic brim. The most likely diagnosis is

a. Multiple myeloma
b. Paget's disease
c. Hypercalcemia
d. Metastatic bone disease

211. The etiology of the process has been shown to be

a. Endocrinopathy
b. Viral infection
c. Malignancy
d. Unknown

212. The treatment of choice for this patient is

a. Observation
b. Nonsteroidal anti-inflammatory
c. Calcitonin or bisphosphonates
d. Interferon α

213. A 50-year-old female is evaluated for hypertension. Her blood pressure is 130/98. She complains of polyuria and of mild muscle weakness. She is on no diuretics or other blood pressure medication. On physical exam, the PMI is displaced to the sixth intercostal space. There is no sign of congestive heart failure and no edema. Laboratory values are as follows:

Na^-: 147 meq/dL
K^-: 2.3 meq/dL
Cl^-: 112 meq/dL
HCO_3: 27 meq/dL

The patient is on no other medication. She does not eat licorice. The first step in diagnosis is

a. 24-h urine for cortisol
b. Urinary metanephrine
c. Plasma renin and aldosterone
d. Renal angiogram

Items 214–216

214. A 40-year-old alcoholic male is being treated for tuberculosis, but he has not been compliant with his medications. He complains of increasing weakness and fatigue. He appears to have lost weight, and his blood pressure is 80/50 mmHg. There is increased pigmentation over the elbows. Cardiac exam is normal. The next step in evaluation should be

a. CBC with iron and iron-binding capacity
b. Erythrocyte sedimentation rate
c. Early morning serum cortisol and cosyntropin stimulation
d. Blood cultures

215. In the advanced stage of this disease, the most likely electrolyte abnormalities will be

a. Low serum Na^+
b. Low serum K^+
c. Low serum Na^+ and high serum K^+
d. Low serum K^+

216. The treatment of choice for this patient is

a. Hydrocortisone once per day
b. Hydrocortisone twice per day plus fludrocortisone
c. Hydrocortisone only during periods of stress
d. Daily ACTH

217. A 60-year-old woman comes to the emergency room in a coma. The patient's temperature is 90°F. She is bradycardic. Her thyroid gland is enlarged. There is bilateral hyporeflexia. The next step in management is

a. Await results of T_4, TSH
b. Obtain T_4, TSH; begin thyroid hormone and glucocorticoid
c. Begin rapid rewarming
d. Obtain CT scan of the head

218. A 19-year old with insulin-dependent diabetes mellitus is taking 30 units of NPH insulin each morning and 15 units at night. Because of persistent morning glycosuria with some ketonuria, the evening dose is increased to 20 units. This worsens the morning glycosuria, and now moderate ketones are noted in urine. The patient complains of sweats and headaches at night. The next step in management is

a. Increase the evening dose of insulin
b. Increase the morning dose of insulin
c. Switch from human NPH to pork insulin
d. Obtain blood sugar levels between 2:00 and 5:00 A.M.

219. A 30-year-old woman is found to have a low serum thyroxine level after being evaluated for fatigue. Five years ago she was treated for Graves' disease with radioactive iodine. The diagnostic test of choice is

a. Serum TSH
b. Serum T_3
c. TRH stimulation test
d. Radioactive iodine uptake

220. A 25-year-old woman is admitted for hypertensive crisis. In the hospital, blood pressure is labile and responds poorly to antihypertensive therapy. The patient complains of palpitations and apprehension. Her past medical history shows that she developed hypotension during an operation for appendicitis.

Hct: 49% (37–48)
WBC: 11 × 10^3 mm (4.3–10.8)
Plasma glucose: 160 mg/dL (75–115)
Plasma calcium: 11 mg/dL (9–10.5)

The most likely diagnosis is

a. Pheochromocytoma
b. Renal artery stenosis
c. Essential hypertension
d. Insulin-dependent diabetes mellitus

Items 221–223

Match each symptom or sign with the appropriate disease.

a. Subacute thyroiditis
b. Graves' disease
c. Surreptitious hyperthyroidism
d. Multinodular goiter
e. Thyroid nodule

221. Weakness, tremor, heat intolerance; raised, thickened skin with peau d'orange appearance **(CHOOSE 1 DISEASE)**

222. Weakness, tremor in male nursing assistant; no ophthalmopathy or skin lesions; RAIU shows subnormal values; T$_4$ elevated **(CHOOSE 1 DISEASE)**

223. Thyroid tender; erythrocyte sedimentation rate elevated; heat intolerance **(CHOOSE 1 DISEASE)**

224. The patient pictured below complains of persistent headache. Her most likely visual field defect is

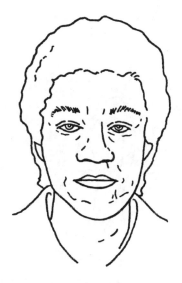

a. Bitemporal hemianopsia
b. Unilateral blindness
c. Left homonymous hemianopsia
d. Right homonymous hemianopsia

225. A patient with small cell carcinoma of the lung develops lethargy. Serum electrolytes are drawn and show a serum sodium of 118 mg/L. There is no evidence of edema, orthostatic hypotension, or dehydration. Urine is concentrated with an osmolality of 320 mmol/kg. Serum BUN, creatinine, and glucose are within normal range. Which of the following is the next appropriate step?

a. Normal saline infusion
b. Diuresis
c. Fluid restriction
d. Tetracycline

226. The 40-year-old woman shown below complains of weakness and amenorrhea. She has hypertension and diabetes mellitus. The clinical findings may be explained by

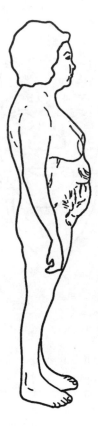

   a. Pituitary tumor
   b. Adrenal tumor
   c. Ectopic ACTH production
   d. Any of the above

227. The patient pictured below presents with gynecomastia and infertility. On exam, he has small, firm testes. Which of the following is correct?

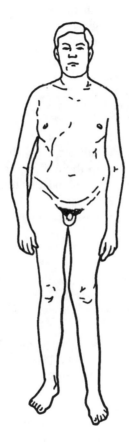

a. The patient is likely to have low levels of gonadotropins
b. The patient has Turner syndrome
c. His most likely karyotype is 47 XXY
d. The patient will have normal sperm count and testosterone level

228. A 52-year-old man complains of impotence. On physical examination, he has an elevated jugular venous pressure, S₃ gallop, and hepatomegaly. He also appears tanned, with pigmentation along joint folds. His left knee is swollen and tender. The plasma glucose is 250 mg/dL, and liver enzymes are elevated. Your next study to establish the diagnosis should be

a. Detection of nocturnal penile tumescence
b. Determination of iron saturation
c. Determination of serum copper
d. Detection of hepatitis B surface antigen
e. Echocardiography

229. A 30-year-old man is evaluated for a thyroid nodule. The patient reports that his father died from thyroid cancer and that a brother had a history of recurrent renal stones. Blood calcitonin concentration is 2000 pg/mL (normal is less than 100); serum calcium and phosphate levels are normal. Before referring the patient to a surgeon, the physician should

a. Obtain a liver scan
b. Perform a calcium infusion test
c. Measure urinary catecholamines
d. Administer suppressive doses of thyroxine and measure levels of thyroid-stimulating hormone
e. Treat the patient with radioactive iodine

230. A 32-year-old woman has a 3-year history of oligomenorrhea that has progressed to amenorrhea during the past year. She has observed loss of breast fullness, reduced hip measurements, acne, increased body hair, and deepening of her voice. Physical examination reveals frontal balding, clitoral hypertrophy, and a male escutcheon. Urinary free cortisol and dehydroepiandrosterone sulfate (DHEAS) are normal. Her plasma testosterone level is 6 ng/mL (normal is 0.2 to 0.8). The most likely diagnosis of this patient's disorder is

a. Cushing syndrome
b. Arrhenoblastoma
c. Polycystic ovary syndrome
d. Granulosa-theca cell tumor

231. A 54-year-old man who has had a Billroth II procedure for peptic ulcer disease now presents with abdominal pain and is found to have recurrent ulcer disease. The physician is considering this patient's illness to be secondary either to a retained antrum or to a gastrinoma. Which of the following tests would best differentiate the two conditions?

a. Random gastrin level
b. Determination of 24-h acid production
c. Serum calcium level
d. Secretin infusion
e. Insulin-induced hypoglycemia

232. A 55-year-old woman who has a history of severe depression and who had radical mastectomy for carcinoma of the breast 1 year previously develops polyuria, nocturia, and excessive thirst. Laboratory values are as follows:

Serum electrolytes: Na⁻ 149 meq/L; K⁻ 3.6 meq/L
Serum calcium: 9.5 mg/dL
Blood glucose: 110 mg/dL
Blood urea nitrogen: 30 mg/dL
Urine osmolality: 150 mOsm/kg

The most likely diagnosis is

a. Psychogenic polydipsia
b. Renal glycosuria
c. Hypercalciuria
d. Diabetes insipidus
e. Inappropriate antidiuretic hormone syndrome

233. A 30-year-old nursing student presents with confusion, sweating, hunger, and fatigue. Blood sugar is noted to be 40 mg/dL. The patient has no history of diabetes mellitus, although her sister is an insulin-dependent diabetic. The patient has had several similar episodes over the past year, all occurring just prior to reporting for work in the early morning. On this evaluation, the patient is found to have high insulin levels and a low C peptide level. The most likely diagnosis is

a. Reactive hypoglycemia
b. Early diabetes mellitus
c. Factitious hypoglycemia
d. Insulinoma

Endocrinology and Metabolic Disease

Answers

195. The answer is b. (*Stobo, 23/e, pp 328–329.*) This obese patient on oral hypoglycemics has developed hyperglycemia and lethargy during an upper respiratory infection. Hyperosmolar nonketotic states that occur in type 2 diabetes can be fatal. When severe hyperglycemia and dehydration increase serum osmolarity above 380 mOsm/L, lethargy or coma occurs. Serum osmolarity is measured by the formula:

$$\frac{\text{Plasma glucose}}{18} + 2\,(\text{serum Na}^+ + \text{K}^+) + \frac{\text{blood urea nitrogen}}{2.8}$$

This patient's serum osmolality is as follows:

$$\frac{(900)}{18} + 2\,(138) + \frac{84}{2.8} = 50 + 276 + 30 = 356$$

Thus the serum osmolality is greater than 350 mOsm/kg. As can be seen from the equation, osmolarity depends mostly on the concentration of sodium. Serum osmolarity will rise significantly when dehydration prevents the dilution of serum sodium that might otherwise occur with hyperglycemia. Hyperosmolarity reflects both hyperglycemia and severe dehydration with hypernatremia. The serum bicarbonate is too high to be consistent with diabetic ketoacidosis. The hyponatremia is related to hyperglycemia. SIADH could not be diagnosed in this clinical setting. Patients with SIADH are not dehydrated but have an inappropriate excretion of ADH that leads to hyponatremia and water retention. The patient's diabetes likely went out of control due to infection. There is no clinical evidence for meningitis.

196. The answer is a. (*Braunwald, 15/e, p 2119.*) The primary treatment for hyperosmolar nonketotic states is fluid replacement, usually normal saline over the first 2 to 3 h. Hypotonic saline may be given for severe hypernatremia or congestive heart failure. Hyperglycemia can be corrected slowly. The patient is not acidotic and would not require bicarbonate treatment (used in severe DKA when pH is less than 7.0). The patient's serum potassium is in the normal range and would not be expected to fall rapidly, but should be monitored.

197. The answer is b. *(Braunwald, 15/e, pp 2114–2116.)* The classification of diabetes mellitus has changed to emphasize the process that leads to hyperglycemia. Type 2 DM is a group of heterogeneous disorders characterized by insulin resistance, impaired secretion of insulin, and increased glucose production. Medical nutrition therapy is a term now used to describe the best possible coordination of calorie intake, weight loss, and exercise. It emphasizes modification of risk factors for hypertension and hyperlipidemia, not just weight loss and calorie restriction. In this type 2 patient, medical nutrition therapy that includes dietary modification, weight loss, and exercise is the first intervention. Blood glucose control should be reevaluated after 3 to 4 weeks. If target blood sugar is not met, pharmacotherapy should be initiated.

198. The answer is b. *(Braunwald, 15/e, pp 2069–2074.)* This patient has clinical symptoms of thyrotoxicosis. Most patients with thyrotoxicosis have increases in total and free concentrations of T_3 and T_4. (Some may have isolated T_3 or T_4 increases.) Most thyrotoxicosis results in suppression of pituitary TSH secretion, so low TSH levels can also confirm the diagnosis.

199. The answer is a. *(Braunwald, 15/e, pp 2069–2074.)* This patient has Graves' disease, which accounts for 60 to 80% of all thyrotoxicosis. In addition to thyrotoxicosis, this patient has orbitopathy as well as the characteristic dermopathy of Graves' disease, called pretibial myxedema. Graves' disease is an autoimmune phenomenon. The extrathyroidal manifestations of the diseases are due to immunologically activated fibroblasts in extraocular muscles and skin. Toxic multinodular goiter produces thyrotoxicosis caused by benign, functionally autonomous tumors. The thyroid gland is usually appreciated as a palpably nodular goiter. Toxic multinodular goiter would not produce the proptosis or dermopathy of Graves' disease. Subacute thyroiditis (de Quervain's) is probably caused by a viral infection. It produces a transient hyperthyroidism followed by hypothyroidism. The thyroid gland is tender.

200. The answer is a. *(Braunwald, 15/e, p 2074.)* Antithyroid drugs are considered by most to be the treatment of choice in a patient with Graves' disease when the underlying illness may remit. Surgical thyroidectomy is usually reserved for those with thyroid malignancy or thyrotoxic pregnant women who have had severe side effects to medication. Surgery complications include hypoparathyroidism and recurrent laryngeal nerve injury. Iodine 131 has been used successfully in Graves' disease and is a reasonable option if the patient is not pregnant or breastfeeding. However, it often causes permanent hypothyroidism. It has also been reported to worsen ophthalmopathy in some patients.

201. The answer is a. *(Braunwald, 15/e, pp 2066–2069.)* This patient presents with classic features of hypothyroidism. Hypothyroidism is almost always caused by autoimmune disease, thyroid damage from surgery, or radiation therapy. Autoimmune thyroiditis usually occurs in women, has a genetic component, and is associated with other autoimmune conditions. Autoimmune thyroiditis may be present with a goiter (Hashimoto's thyroiditis) or with minimal residual thyroid tissue (atrophic thyroiditis). Primary hypothyroidism can result from surgery or radiation therapy, but there is no such history in this patient. Thyroid cancer does not cause hypothyroidism. It presents with neck mass, hoarse voice, or expanding nodule.

202. The answer is a. *(Braunwald, 15/e, p 2068.)* Once hypothyroidism is diagnosed by clinical features, TSH and free T_4 measurements, etiology can be confirmed by measuring the presence of autoantibody—particularly thyroid peroxidase (TPO), which is present in 90 to 95% of patients with autoimmune hypothyroidism. Biopsy by fine needle aspirate can confirm the diagnosis but is not necessary in most cases.

203. The answer is d. *(Braunwald, 15/e, p 2083.)* Palpable thyroid nodules are common, occurring in about 5% of all adults. Thyroid fine needle biopsy now plays a central role in the differential diagnosis of thyroid nodules. If the TSH is normal, as it is in this patient, then fine needle aspirate biopsy is indicated and will distinguish cysts from benign lesions or neoplasms. In about 14% of such cases, biopsy will be suspicious or diagnostic for malignancy and surgery will be necessary. Thyroid scan can show a hot nodule, which would be reassuring that the nodule is benign; however, a biopsy would be necessary for cold nodules. Thyroid sonography seldom can rule out malignancy in palpable nodules.

204–206. The answers are 204-c, 205-b, 206-d. *(Braunwald, 15/e, pp 2032–2052.)* Cushing's disease produces hypercortisolism secondary to excessive excretion of pituitary ACTH. It often affects women in their childbearing years. Cervical fat pad, purple striae, and hirsutism are characteristic features, as well as muscle wasting, easy bruising, amenorrhea, and psychiatric disturbances. Prolactinoma, or prolactin-secreting adenoma, may cause bitemporal hemianopsia—as all pituitary tumors can. Galactorrhea (lactation not associated with pregnancy) and irregular menses or amenorrhea are the clinical clues. Serum prolactin levels are usually over 250 ng/mL, often distinguishing them from other causes of hyperprolactinemia such as renal failure. Empty sella syndrome is enlargement of the sella turcica from CSF pressure compressing the pituitary gland. It is likely to occur in obese, hypertensive women. There are no focal findings. Some patients have chronic headaches; others are asymptomatic. MRI will distinguish this syndrome from a pituitary tumor. These patients have normal pituitary function, the rim of pituitary tissue being fully functional.

207. The answer is d. *(Braunwald, 15/e, p 2128.)* An active lifestyle and good exercise program can prevent the complications of diabetes. Benefits include blood pressure control, reduction in body fat, weight loss, and increased insulin sensitivity. However, there are pitfalls to such a program. Some forms of exercise might jeopardize adequate foot care, and foot exam becomes particularly important in the patient who is doing weight-bearing exercise. Exercise can induce hypoglycemia by potentiating insulin action; this is particularly true in the type 1 diabetic. Diabetics who have risk factors for cardiovascular disease, such as hypertension and hyperlipidemia, should undergo an exercise stress test prior to engaging in a rigorous exercise program. This is important because asymptomatic cardiovascular disease is more common in diabetics.

208. The answer is c. *(Braunwald, 15/e, p 2128.)* In order to reduce plasma cholesterol and decrease the risk of vascular disease, fat intake should be moderated, with less than 10% of total caloric intake being saturated fat. Caloric distribution does not restrict or decrease carbohydrates. Use of caloric sweeteners, including sucrose, is acceptable as long as it is matched to insulin demand. Dietary protein should provide 10 to 20% of total calories. In patients with diabetic nephropathy, reducing dietary protein to 10% is often recommended. Caloric intake is not consistent from day to day but is matched with level of activity.

209. The answer is c. (*Braunwald, 15/e, pp 292–294.*) The first step in the evaluation of impotence is a complete and detailed history, including libido and ability to attain erection unrelated to sexual intercourse. Loss of all erectile function suggests an organic cause for the disease. In this patient, impotence may be the result of depression from the antihypertensive agent or a direct effect of the beta blocker on sexual performance. Diabetes may cause impotence as an effect on penile blood supply or parasympathetic nervous system function. A decrease in libido would suggest testosterone deficiency. Serum testosterone should then be measured, and, if low, serum gonadotropins should be measured. In a diabetic with claudication or abnormal femoral pulses, injection of papaverine into the corpora cavernosa can test vascular insufficiency as the cause of impotence. A normal response is an erection within 10 min.

210. The answer is b. (*Braunwald, 15/e, pp 2237–2239.*) This patient has widespread Paget's disease of bone. Excessive resorption of bone is followed by replacement of normal marrow with dense, trabecular, disorganized bone. Hearing loss and tinnitus are due to direct involvement of the ossicles of the inner ear. Plasma alkaline phosphatase levels represent increased bone turnover. Neither myeloma or metastatic bone disease would result in bony deformity such as skull enlargement. Alkaline phosphatase is a marker of bone formation and does not rise in pure lytic lesions such as multiple myeloma.

211. The answer is d. (*Braunwald, 15/e, p 2237.*) The cause of Paget's disease remains unknown. Some intranuclear inclusions resemble the nucleocapsids of viruses. Measles and respiratory syncytial virus mRNA appears similar to mRNA found in nucleocapsids. No known endocrinopathy has been suggested, and Paget's disease does not involve malignant cells. There is increasing interest in a genetic predisposition for the disease, and some kindreds have an autosomal dominant inheritance pattern.

212. The answer is c. *(Braunwald, 15/e, p 2239.)* Most patients with Paget's disease do not require treatment as they are asymptomatic. Bone pain, hearing loss, bony deformity, congestive heart failure, hypercalcemia, and repeated fractures are all indications for specific therapy beyond just the symptomatic relief of nonsteroidal anti-inflammatory agents. Calcitonin restores normal bone modeling. Bisphosphonates bind to hydroxyapatite crystals to decrease bone turnover. Bisphosphonates are now generally recommended as the treatment of choice. Newer bisphosphonates such as alendronate have replaced editronate because they are more potent and do not produce mineralization defects. Calcitonin is still used in patients who cannot tolerate the GI side effects of alendronate.

213. The answer is c. *(Braunwald, 15/e, pp 2095–2096.)* The patient has diastolic hypertension with associated hypokalemia. She is not taking diuretics. There is no edema on physical exam. Excessive inappropriate aldosterone production will produce a hypertension with hypokalemia syndrome. Hypersecretion of aldosterone increases distal tubular exchange of sodium for potassium with progressive depletion of body potassium. The hypertension is due to increased sodium absorption. Very low plasma renin that fails to increase with appropriate stimulus (such as volume depletion) and hypersecretion of aldosterone suggest the diagnosis of primary hyperaldosteronism. Suppressed renin activity occurs in about 25% of hypertensive patients with essential hypertension. Lack of suppression of aldosterone is also necessary to diagnose primary aldosteronism. High aldosterone levels that are not suppressed by saline loading prove that there is a primary inappropriate secretion of aldosterone. A 24-h urine for free cortisol would be used in the workup of a patient with Cushing syndrome. Urinary metanephrine is a screening test for pheochromocytoma.

214. The answer is c. *(Braunwald, 15/e, pp 2098–2099.)* This patient's symptoms of weakness, fatigue, and weight loss in combination with signs of hypotension and extensor hyperpigmentation are all consistent with Addison's disease (adrenal insufficiency). Tuberculosis can involve the adrenal glands and result in adrenal insufficiency. Measurement of serum cortisol baseline and then stimulation with ACTH will confirm the clinical suspicion. The ACTH stimulation test is used to determine the adrenal reserve capacity for steroid production. Cortisol response is measured 60 min after cosyntropin is given intramuscularly or intravenously.

215. The answer is c. *(Braunwald, 15/e, pp 2098–2099.)* Hyponatremia is due to loss of sodium in the urine (aldosterone deficiency) and movement of sodium intracellularly. Extravascular sodium loss causes hypotension. Hyperkalemia is due to aldosterone deficiency, impaired glomerular filtration, and acidosis.

216. The answer is b. *(Braunwald, 15/e, pp 2098–2099.)* Hydrocortisone is the mainstay of treatment. Two-thirds of the dose is taken in the morning and one-third at night in order to approach normal diurnal variation. The recommended dose is 20 to 30 mg/d. The mineralocorticoid component of adrenal hormones also needs to be replaced. Fludrocortisone is given at a dosage of 0.05 to 0.1 mg/d. During periods of intercurrent stress or illness, higher doses of both glucocorticoid and mineralocorticoid are required.

217. The answer is b. *(Braunwald, 15/e, p 2069.)* The clinical concern in this patient is myxedema coma. Once this diagnosis is considered, treatment must be started, as it is a medical emergency. Treatment is initiated; should lab results not support the diagnosis, then treatment would be stopped. An intravenous bolus of thyroxine is given (300 to 500 µg), followed by daily intravenous doses. Glucocorticoids are given concomitantly. Intravenous fluids are also needed; rewarming should be accompanied slowly, so as not to precipitate cardiac arrhythmias. If alveolar ventilation is compromised, then intubation may also be necessary.

218. The answer is d. *(Stein, 5/e, p 1861.)* Episodic hypoglycemia at night is followed by rebound hyperglycemia. This condition, called the Somogyi phenomenon, develops in response to excessive insulin administration. An adrenergic response to hypoglycemia results in increased glycogenolysis, gluconeogenesis, and diminished glucose uptake by peripheral tissues. After hypoglycemia is documented, the insulin dosages are slowly reduced.

219. The answer is a. *(Stein, 5/e, pp 1808–1811.)* TSH levels are always increased in patients with untreated hypothyroidism (from primary thyroid disease) and would be the test of choice in this patient. Serum T_3 is not sensitive for hypothyroidism. The TRH stimulation test is used to assess pituitary reserve of thyroid-stimulating hormone. A decreased RAIU is of limited value because of the low value for the lower limit of normal. In goitrous hypothyroidism, the RAIU may even be increased.

220. The answer is a. *(Braunwald, 15/e, pp 2105–2106.)* A hypertensive crisis in this young woman suggests a secondary cause of hypertension. In the setting of palpitations, apprehension, and hyperglycemia, pheochromocytoma should be considered. Pheochromocytomas are derived from the adrenal medulla. They are capable of producing and secreting catecholamines. Unexplained hypotension associated with surgery or trauma may also suggest the disease. Clinical symptoms are the result of catecholamine secretion. For example, the patient's hyperglycemia is a result of a catecholamine effect of insulin suppression and stimulation of hepatic glucose output. Hypercalcemia has been attributed to ectopic secretion of parathormone-related protein. Renal artery stenosis can cause severe hypertension but would not explain the systemic symptoms or laboratory abnormalities in this case.

221–223. The answers are 221-b, 222-c, 223-a. *(Braunwald, 15/e, pp 2069–2075.)* Symptoms of hyperthyroidism with skin involvement characteristic of pretibial myxedema suggest Graves' disease. Skin and eye involvement in association with hyperthyroid symptoms do not occur in hyperthyroidism other than Graves' disease. Surreptitious hyperthyroidism can occur in health care workers who have access to thyroid hormone. Classic symptoms of hyperthyroidism occur and the serum T_4 is elevated. Radioactive iodine uptake would show subnormal values, as there is no increased thyroid uptake in the gland itself. The thyroid gland is not palpable. A tender thyroid gland and elevated ESR make subacute thyroiditis a likely diagnosis. Hyperthyroid symptoms are common early in the illness.

224. The answer is a. *(Braunwald, 15/e, pp 2045–2046.)* The patient shows excessive growth of soft tissue that has resulted in coarsening of facial features, prognathism, and frontal bossing—all characteristic of acromegaly. This growth hormone–secreting pituitary tumor will result in bitemporal hemianopsia when the tumor impinges on the optic chiasm, which lies just above the sella turcica.

225. The answer is c. *(Braunwald, 15/e, pp 2058–2059.)* The patient described has hyponatremia, normovolemia, and concentrated urine. These features are sufficient to make a diagnosis of inappropriate antidiuretic hormone secretion. Inappropriate ADH secretion occurs, in some cases, due to ectopic production by neoplastic tissue. Treatment necessitates restriction of fluid intake. A negative water balance results in a rise in serum Na^+ and serum osmolality and symptom improvement. This syndrome can occur as a side effect of many drugs or from carcinoma, head trauma, infections, neurologic diseases, or stroke.

226. The answer is d. *(Braunwald, 15/e, pp 2091–2093.)* The clinical findings all suggest an excess production of cortisol by the adrenal gland. Hypertension, truncal obesity, and abdominal striae are common physical findings. The process responsible for continued excess could be any of those listed—an ACTH-secreting pituitary tumor, an ectopic ACTH-producing neoplasm, or a primary adrenal tumor.

227. The answer is c. *(Braunwald, 15/e, pp 2173–2174.)* The picture of infertility, gynecomastia, and tall stature is consistent with Klinefelter syndrome and an XXY karyotype. The patient has abnormal gonadal development with hyalinized testes that result in low testosterone levels and elevated levels of gonadotropin. Turner syndrome refers to the 45 karyotype that results in abnormal sexual development in a female.

228. The answer is b. *(Braunwald, 15/e, pp 2257–2260.)* Iron overload should be considered among patients who present with any one or a combination of the following: hepatomegaly, weakness, pigmentation, atypical arthritis, diabetes, impotence, unexplained chronic abdominal pain, or cardiomyopathy. Excessive alcohol intake increases the diagnostic probability. Diagnostic suspicions should be particularly high when the family history is positive for similar clinical findings. The most frequent cause of iron overload is a common genetic disorder known as (idiopathic) hemochromatosis. Secondary iron storage problems can occur in a variety of anemias. The most practical screening test is the determination of serum iron, transferrin saturation, and plasma ferritin. Plasma ferritin values above 300 ng/mL in males and 200 ng/mL in females suggest increased iron stores. Genetic screening is now used to assess which patients are at risk for severe fibrosis of the liver. Definitive diagnosis can be established by liver biopsy. Determination of serum copper is needed when Wilson's disease is the probable cause of hepatic abnormalities. The clinical picture here is inconsistent with that diagnosis. Nocturnal penile tumescence and echocardiogram can confirm clinical findings but will not help to establish the diagnosis.

229. The answer is c. (*Braunwald, 15/e, p 2187.*) For the patient described, the markedly increased calcitonin levels indicate the diagnosis of medullary carcinoma of the thyroid. In view of the family history, the patient most likely has multiple endocrine neoplasia (MEN) type II, which includes medullary carcinoma of the thyroid gland, pheochromocytoma, and parathyroid hyperplasia. Pheochromocytoma may exist without sustained hypertension, as indicated by excessive urinary catecholamines. Before thyroid surgery is performed on this patient, a pheochromocytoma must be ruled out through urinary catecholamine determinations; the presence of such a tumor might expose him to a hypertensive crisis during surgery. The entire thyroid gland must be removed because foci of parafollicular cell hyperplasia, a premalignant lesion, may be scattered throughout the gland. Successful removal of the medullary carcinoma can be monitored with serum calcitonin levels. Hyperparathyroidism, while unlikely in this patient, is probably present in his brother. Hypoparathyroidism is unlikely with a normal serum calcium level.

230. The answer is b. (*Braunwald, 15/e, p 300.*) The symptoms of masculinization (e.g., alopecia, deepening of voice, clitoral hypertrophy) in the patient presented in the question are characteristic of active androgen-producing tumors. Such extreme virilization is very rarely observed in polycystic ovary syndrome or in Cushing syndrome; moreover, the presence of normal cortisol and markedly elevated plasma testosterone levels indicates an ovarian rather than adrenal cause of the findings. Arrhenoblastomas are the most common androgen-producing ovarian tumors. Their incidence is highest during the reproductive years. Composed of varying proportions of Leydig's and Sertoli cells, they are generally benign. In contrast to arrhenoblastomas, granulosa-theca cell tumors produce feminization, not virilization.

231. The answer is d. (*Braunwald, 15/e, pp 595–599, 1661–1662.*) The diagnosis of gastrinoma should be considered in all patients with recurrent ulcers after surgical correction for peptic ulcer disease, ulcers in the distal duodenum or jejunum, ulcer disease associated with diarrhea, or evidence suggestive of the multiple endocrine neoplasia (MEN) type I (familial association of pituitary, parathyroid, and pancreatic tumors) in ulcer patients. Because basal serum gastrin and basal acid production may both be normal or only slightly elevated in patients with gastrinomas, provocative tests may be needed for diagnosis. Both the secretin and calcium infusion tests are used; a paradoxical increase in serum gastrin concentration is seen in response to both infusions in patients with gastrinomas. In contrast, other conditions associated with hypergastrinemia, such as duodenal ulcers, retained antrum, gastric outlet obstruction, antral G cell hyperplasia, and pernicious anemia, will respond with either no change or a decrease in serum gastrin.

232. The answer is d. (*Braunwald, 15/e, p 2054–2056.*) Metastatic tumors rarely cause diabetes insipidus, but of the tumors that may cause it, carcinoma of the breast is by far the most common. In this patient, the diagnosis of diabetes insipidus is suggested by hypernatremia and low urine osmolality. Psychogenic polydipsia is an unlikely diagnosis since serum sodium is usually mildly reduced in this condition. Renal glycosuria would be expected to induce a higher urine osmolality than this patient has because of the osmotic effect of glucose. While nephrocalcinosis secondary to hypercalcemia may produce polyuria, hypercalciuria does not. Finally, the findings of inappropriate antidiuretic hormone syndrome are the opposite of those observed in diabetes insipidus and thus are incompatible with the clinical picture in this patient.

233. The answer is c. (*Braunwald, 15/e, pp. 2138–2142.*) This clinical picture and laboratory results suggest factitious hypoglycemia caused by self-administration of insulin. The diagnosis should be suspected in health care workers, patients or family members with diabetes, and others who have a history of malingering. Patients present with symptoms of hypoglycemia and low plasma glucose levels. Insulin levels will be high, but without a concomitant rise in C peptide. Endogenous hyperinsulinism, such as would be seen with an insulinoma, would result in elevated plasma insulin concentrations (>36 pmol/L) and elevated C peptide levels (>0.2 mmol/L). C peptide is derived from the breakdown of proinsulin, which is produced endogenously; thus C peptide will not rise in the patient who develops hypoglycemia from exogenous insulin. Reactive hypoglycemia occurs after meals and is self-limited. A rapid postprandial rise in glucose may induce a brisk insulin response that causes transient hypoglycemia hours later. It may be associated with gastric or intestinal surgery.

Gastroenterology

Questions

DIRECTIONS: Each item below contains a question or incomplete statement followed by suggested responses. Select the **one best** response to each question.

234. A 35-year-old alcoholic male is admitted for nausea, vomiting, and abdominal pain that radiates to the back. The laboratory value that suggests a poor prognosis in this patient is

a. Elevated serum lipase
b. Elevated serum amylase
c. Leukocytosis of 20,000/μm
d. Diastolic blood pressure greater than 90 mmHg

DIRECTIONS: Each group of questions below consists of lettered options followed by a set of numbered items. For each numbered item, select the **one** lettered option with which it is **most** closely associated. Each lettered option may be used once, more than once, or not at all.

Items 235–237

Match the patient described with the most likely diagnosis.

a. Acute diverticulitis
b. Acute pancreatitis
c. Acute cholecystitis
d. Intestinal obstruction
e. Irritable bowel syndrome

235. A 45-year-old moderately obese white woman presents with four episodes of severe epigastric and right upper quadrant pain, each episode lasting 30 to 60 min and accompanied by nausea and vomiting. Her most recent episode was very severe, with the pain radiating to the inferior angle of the scapula. **(CHOOSE 1 DIAGNOSIS)**

236. A 78-year-old white man presents with a 3-day history of gradually worsening left lower quadrant pain. He does not have rectal bleeding or weight loss but has noticed mild constipation in association with the pain. He has a temperature of 100.2°F, moderate left lower quadrant tenderness without evidence of peritoneal inflammation, and a white count of 14,200. **(CHOOSE 1 DIAGNOSIS)**

237. A 68-year-old woman who has had a previous open cholecystectomy presents with an 8-h history of cramping periumbilical pain. Each episode of pain lasts 3 to 5 min and then abates. Over several hours she develops nausea, vomiting, and abdominal distension. She has been unable to pass stool or flatus for the past 4 h. **(CHOOSE 1 DIAGNOSIS)**

Items 238–240

238. A 40-year-old cigarette smoker complains of epigastric pain, well localized, nonradiating, and described as burning. The pain is partially relieved by eating. There is no weight loss. He has not used nonsteroidal anti-inflammatory agents. The pain has gradually worsened over several months. The most sensitive way to make a specific diagnosis is

a. Barium x-ray
b. Endoscopy
c. Serologic test for *Helicobacter pylori*
d. Serum gastrin

239. The patient is found to have a duodenal ulcer by upper endoscopy. The likelihood of this patient having *H. pylori* in the gastric antrum is

a. 5%
b. 10%
c. 30 to 60%
d. 100%

240. The best way to eradicate *H. pylori* in this patient is

a. Omeprazole 20 mg PO daily for 6 weeks
b. Ranitidine 300 mg PO qhs for 6 weeks
c. Omeprazole 20 mg BID, amoxicillin 1000 mg BID, clarithromycin 500 mg BID for 14 days
d. Pepto-Bismol and metronidazole BID for 7 days
e. Sulcrafate 200 μg QID for 6 weeks

Items 241–242

241. A 70-year-old male presents with a complaint of fatigue. There is no history of alcohol abuse or liver disease; the patient is on no medication. Scleral icterus is noted on physical exam. There is no evidence for chronic liver disease on physical exam, and the liver and spleen are nonpalpable. The patient is noted to have a normocytic, normochromic anemia. The first step in evaluation of this patient is

a. CT scan of the abdomen
b. Hepatitis profile
c. Liver function tests, including direct versus indirect bilirubin and urine bilirubin
d. Abdominal ultrasound

242. The patient above is noted to have conjugated hyperbilirubinema, with bilirubin detected in the urine. Serum bilirubin is 12 mg/dL, AST and ALT are in normal range, and alkaline phosphatase is 300 U/L (3 times normal). The next step in evaluation is

a. Ultrasound or CT scan
b. Hepatitis profile
c. Reticulocyte count
d. Family history for hemochromatosis

Items 243–245

243. A 40-year-old male with long-standing alcohol abuse complains of abdominal swelling, which has been progressive over several months. He has a history of gastrointestinal bleeding. On physical exam, there are spider angiomas and palmar erythema. Abdominal collateral vessels are seen around the umbilicus. There is shifting dullness, and bulging flanks are noted. An important first step in the patient's evaluation is

a. Diagnostic paracentesis
b. UGI series
c. Ethanol level
d. CT scan

244. A paracentesis is performed on the patient previously described. The serum albumin minus ascitic fluid albumin equals 1.4 g/dL. The most likely diagnosis is

a. Portal hypertension
b. Pancreatitis
c. Tuberculous peritonitis
d. Hepatoma

245. While hospitalized, the patient's mental status deteriorates. He has been having guaiac-positive stools and a low-grade fever. He has also received sedation for agitation. On physical exam, the patient is confused. He has no meningeal signs and no focal neurologic findings. There is hyperreflexia and a nonrhythmic flapping tremor of the wrist. The most likely explanation for the mental status change is

a. Tuberculosis meningitis
b. Subdural hematoma
c. Alcohol withdrawal seizure
d. Hepatic encephalopathy

246. A 50-year-old black male with a history of alcohol and tobacco abuse has complained of difficulty swallowing solid food for the past 2 months. More recently, swallowing fluids has also become a problem. He has noted black, tarry stools on occasion. The patient has lost 10 lb. Which of the following statements is correct?

a. The patient's prognosis is good
b. Barium contrast study is indicated
c. The most likely diagnosis is peptic ulcer disease
d. The patient has achalasia

247. A 34-year-old male presents with substernal discomfort. The symptoms are worse after meals, particularly a heavy evening meal, and are sometimes associated with hot/sour fluid in the back of the throat and nocturnal awakening. The patient denies difficulty swallowing, pain on swallowing, or weight loss. The symptoms have been present for 6 weeks; the patient has gained 20 lb in the past 2 years. Your initial approach is

a. A therapeutic trial of ranitidine
b. Exercise test with thallium imaging
c. Esophagogastroduodenoscopy
d. CT scan of the chest

248. A 48-year-old woman presents with a change in bowel habits and 10-lb weight loss despite preservation of appetite. She notices increased abdominal gas, particularly after fatty meals. The stools are malodorous and occur 2 to 3 times per day; no rectal bleeding is noticed. The symptoms are less prominent when the patient follows a clear liquid diet. The most likely histological abnormality associated with this patient's symptoms is

a. Signet ring cells on gastric biopsy
b. Mucosal inflammation and crypt abscesses on sigmoidoscopy
c. Villous atrophy and increased lymphocytes in the lamina propria on small bowel biopsy
d. Small, curved gram-negative bacteria in areas of intestinal metaplasia on gastric biopsy

249. A nursing student has just completed her hepatitis B vaccine series. On reviewing her laboratory studies (assuming she has no prior exposure to hepatitis B), you expect

a. Positive test for hepatitis B surface antigen
b. Antibody against hepatitis B surface antigen (anti-HBS) alone
c. Antibody against hepatitis core antigen (anti-HBC)
d. Antibody against both surface and core antigen
e. Antibody against hepatitis E antigen

Items 250–252

Match the clinical description with the most likely disease process.

a. Primary biliary cirrhosis
b. Sclerosing cholangitis
c. Anaerobic liver abscess
d. Hepatoma
e. Hepatitis C
f. Hepatitis D
g. Hemochromatosis

250. A 40-year-old white female complains of pruritus. She has an elevated alkaline phosphatase and positive antimitochondrial antibody test. **(CHOOSE 1 DISEASE PROCESS)**

251. A 70-year-old male with a long history of diverticulitis has low-grade fever, elevated alkaline phosphatase, and right upper quadrant pain. **(CHOOSE 1 DISEASE PROCESS)**

252. A 30-year-old male with ulcerative colitis develops jaundice, pruritus, and right upper quadrant pain. Liver biopsy shows an inflammatory obliterative process affecting intrahepatic and extrahepatic bile ducts. **(CHOOSE 1 DISEASE PROCESS)**

253. A 40-year-old male has a history of three duodenal ulcers with prompt recurrence. Symptoms have been associated with severe diarrhea. One of the ulcers occurred close to the jejunum. Serum gastrin levels have been 200 pg/mL. The most useful test in this patient is

a. Colonoscopy
b. Endoscopic retrograde cholangiogram
c. CT scan of abdomen
d. Secretin injection test
e. Upper gastrointestinal series

254. A 40-year-old white male complains of weakness, weight loss, and abdominal pain. On examination, the patient has diffuse hyperpigmentation and a palpable liver edge. Polyarthritis of the wrists and hips is also noted. Fasting blood sugar is 185 mg/dL. The most likely diagnosis is

a. Insulin-dependent diabetes mellitus
b. Pancreatic carcinoma
c. Addison's disease
d. Hemochromatosis

Items 255–257

Match the clinical description with the most likely disease process.

a. Hemolysis secondary to G6PD deficiency
b. Pancreatic carcinoma
c. Acute viral hepatitis
d. Crigler-Najjar syndrome
e. Gilbert syndrome
f. Cirrhosis of liver

255. An African American male develops mild jaundice while being treated for a urinary tract infection. Urine bilirubin is negative. Serum bilirubin is 3 mg/dL, all unconjugated. Hemoglobin is 7. **(CHOOSE 1 DISEASE PROCESS)**

256. A 60-year-old male is noted to have mild jaundice and weight loss. Alkaline phosphatase is very elevated. The patient has had very pale stools. **(CHOOSE 1 DISEASE PROCESS)**

257. A young woman complains of fatigue, change in skin color, and dark brown urine. She has right upper quadrant tenderness and ALT of 1035 (normal is 8 to 20). **(CHOOSE 1 DISEASE PROCESS)**

258. A 32-year-old white woman complains of abdominal pain off and on since the age of 17. She notices abdominal bloating relieved by defecation as well as alternating diarrhea and constipation. She has no weight loss, GI bleeding, or nocturnal diarrhea. On examination, she has slight LLQ tenderness and gaseous abdominal distension. Laboratory studies, including CBC, are normal. Your initial approach should be

a. Recommend increased dietary fiber, prn antispasmodics, and follow-up exam in 2 months
b. Refer to gastroenterologist for colonoscopy
c. Obtain antiendomysial antibodies
d. Order UGI series with small bowel follow-through

259. A 55-year-old white woman has had recurrent episodes of alcohol-induced pancreatitis. Despite abstinence, the patient develops postprandial abdominal pain, bloating, weight loss despite good appetite, and bulky, foul-smelling stools. KUB shows pancreatic calcifications. In this patient, you expect

a. Diabetes mellitus
b. Malabsorption of fat-soluble vitamins D and K
c. Guaiac-positive stool
d. Courvoisier's sign

260. A 34-year-old white woman is treated for a UTI with amoxicillin. Initially she improves, but 5 days after beginning treatment, she develops recurrent fever, abdominal bloating, and diarrhea with six to eight loose stools per day. You suspect antibiotic-associated colitis. The best diagnostic test is

a. Identification of *Clostridium difficile* toxin in the stool
b. Isolation of *C. difficile* in a stool culture
c. Stool positive for white blood cells
d. Detection of IgG antibodies against *C. difficile* in the serum

Items 261–264

For each case scenario, suggest the most likely diagnosis.

a. Gastric ulcer
b. Aortoenteric fistula
c. Mallory-Weiss tear
d. Esophageal varices
e. Hereditary hemorrhagic telangiectasia (HHT)

261. An 88-year-old white woman is taking naproxen for osteoarthritis. She has noticed mild epigastric discomfort for several weeks, but has continued the naproxen because of improvement in joint symptoms. She suddenly develops hematemesis and hypotension. **(CHOOSE 1 DIAGNOSIS)**

262. A 42-year-old white woman with a history of alcohol abuse develops nausea and vomiting without abdominal pain. After several bouts of retching, she vomits bright red blood. Physical exam is negative, without spider angiomata or splenomegaly. LFTs are normal. **(CHOOSE 1 DIAGNOSIS)**

263. A 76-year-old white man presents with painless hematemesis and hypotension. He has no previous GI symptoms but did have resection of an abdominal aortic aneurysm 12 years previously. EGD shows no bleeding source in the stomach or duodenum. **(CHOOSE 1 DIAGNOSIS)**

264. A 23-year-old man develops iron-deficiency anemia and heme-positive stools. His weight is stable. A few telangiectasias are present on the lips. Abdominal exam is negative without hepatosplenomegaly. **(CHOOSE 1 DIAGNOSIS)**

Items 265–268

For each case scenario, suggest the likeliest diagnosis.

a. Ulcerative colitis
b. Crohn's disease
c. Ischemic colitis
d. Diverticulitis
e. Amebic colitis

265. A 32-year-old white female presents with a 3-week history of diarrhea with the passage of blood and mucus. Sigmoidoscopy shows inflamed, friable mucosa from rectum to midsigmoid. Proximal involvement is not seen. Biopsy reveals inflammation with crypt abscesses. **(CHOOSE 1 DIAGNOSIS)**

266. A 35-year-old white man presents with diarrhea, weight loss, and RLQ pain. On exam, a tender mass is noted in the RLQ; the stool is guaiac-positive. Colonoscopy shows segmental areas of inflammation. SBFT shows nodular thickening of the terminal ileum. **(CHOOSE 1 DIAGNOSIS)**

267. A 75-year-old African American woman, previously healthy, presents with low-grade fever, diarrhea, and rectal bleeding. Colonoscopy shows continuous erythema from rectum to mid–transverse colon. The cecum is normal. **(CHOOSE 1 DIAGNOSIS)**

268. A 70-year-old white woman presents with LLQ abdominal pain, low-grade fever, and mild rectal bleeding. Examination shows LLQ tenderness. Unprepped sigmoidoscopy reveals segmental inflammation beginning in the distal sigmoid colon through the mid–descending colon. The rest of the exam is negative. **(CHOOSE 1 DIAGNOSIS)**

Items 269–272

For each of the following case scenarios, suggest the likeliest pathogen.

a. *Staphylococcus aureus*
b. *Shigella dysenteriae*
c. *Entamoeba histolytica*
d. *Giardia lamblia*
e. *Yersinia enterocolitica*

269. A 21-year-old white male presents with 10-lb weight loss, abdominal bloating, and bulky, loose stools. He has no history of travel, but he does drink from a surface water source. **(CHOOSE 1 PATHOGEN)**

270. A 44-year-old Hispanic man recently immigrated from Mexico. Beginning 2 weeks before the move, he developed lower abdominal pain, weight loss, and bloody, mucusy stools. **(CHOOSE 1 PATHOGEN)**

271. Two hours after ingesting potato salad at a picnic, a 50-year-old white woman develops severe nausea and vomiting. She has no diarrhea, fever, or chills. On exam, she appears hypovolemic, but the abdomen is benign. **(CHOOSE 1 PATHOGEN)**

272. A 30-year-old day care worker develops profuse bloody diarrhea, abdominal pain, and fever to 104°F. Exam reveals mild lower abdominal tenderness without rebound. WBC is 23,000. Several schoolchildren have had a similar illness. **(CHOOSE 1 PATHOGEN)**

Gastroenterology

Answers

234. The answer is c. (*Braunwald, 15/e, pp 1793–1799.*) The Ranson criteria are used to determine prognosis in acute pancreatitis. Factors that adversely affect survival include age greater than 55 years, leukocytosis greater than 16,000/μm, glucose greater than 200 mg/dL, LDH greater than 400 IU, and AST greater than 250 IU/L. After the initial 48 h, a fall in hematocrit, hypocalcemia, hypoxemia, an increase in BUN, and hypoalbuminemia are also poor prognostic findings. Hypotension with systolic BP less than 90 mmHg is also a poor prognostic sign; diastolic hypertension is not correlated with prognosis.

235–237. The answers are 235-c, 236-a, 237-d. (*Braunwald, 15/e, pp 1695–1696, 1703–1705, 1776–1784.*) Most gallstones are asymptomatic (about 15% of patients with incidentally discovered gallstones develop symptoms after 10 years). Symptoms of gallstones are usually caused by passage of a small stone down the cystic and common bile duct. While the stone is in the duct, it causes somewhat poorly localized visceral pain that is most often felt in the epigastrium or right upper quadrant. Usually the stone passes and the episode of biliary colic resolves after 30 to 60 min. If the stone becomes lodged in the cystic duct, acute cholecystitis develops. Acute inflammation causes distension and inflammation of the gallbladder, which then irritates the nerves of the parietal peritoneum. Then the pain becomes clearly localized to the right upper quadrant, becomes constant, and is associated with right upper quadrant tenderness and pain on inspiration (leading to Murphy's sign or respiratory arrest on palpation in the right upper quadrant).

Diverticula of the colon are also usually asymptomatic. Over 50% of patients above the age of 70 years will be shown to have diverticula by barium enema or colonoscopy. Symptoms of acute diverticulitis occur when microscopic perforation of the thin wall of the diverticular sac causes abdominal pain. Since diverticula are 3 times as common in the left colon as in the right, most acute diverticulitis is associated with left lower quadrant pain. Tenderness over the sigmoid colon is associated with mild peritoneal inflammation, low-grade fever, and leukocytosis. Evidence of generalized peritonitis is rare. Patients at this stage are usually managed with oral antibiotics; intravenous antibiotics are used if the patient suffers from vomiting or is severely ill. Antibiotics that cover usual colonic flora (gram-negative rods and anaerobes) will normally lead to resolution of diverticulitis. Diagnostic studies are generally deferred for several weeks for fear of worsening diverticulitis or causing perforation.

Acute intestinal obstruction is most often associated with adhesive bands from previous surgery. Hysterectomy and appendectomy are the most common preceding surgeries, although any operation associated with entry into the peritoneum can cause adhesions. The patient usually has the classic colicky pain associated with several pain-free minutes before the pain again builds up to maximum intensity. This kind of pain is much more commonly associated with intestinal obstruction than biliary or renal disease (so-called biliary and renal colic are often constant pains).

238. The answer is b. (*Braunwald, 15/e, pp 1649–1661.*) Localized epigastric burning pain relieved by eating requires evaluation for peptic ulcer disease. Upper gastrointestinal endoscopy provides the best sensitivity and specificity; barium swallow is less expensive, but is less accurate in defining mucosal disease. Patients with refractory or recurrent disease should have serum gastrin levels measured to rule out gastrinoma. A positive antibody test for *H. pylori* would only indicate previous exposure.

239. The answer is c. (*Braunwald, 15/e, pp 1652–1654.*) *H. pylori* is present in 30 to 60% of patients who have a duodenal ulcer not associated with NSAID ingestion. In gastric ulcer, the incidence of *H. pylori* is higher (70%). *H. pylori* is more common in developing countries and in patients with low socioeconomic status, in particular those with unsanitary living conditions, which suggests that *H. pylori* is transmitted by fecal-oral or oral-oral routes. Before the discovery of *H. pylori*, most duodenal ulcers would reoccur.

240. The answer is c. (*Braunwald, 15/e, pp 1652–1654.*) Although acid suppression therapy leads to 80% healing rates after 4 weeks of treatment, acid reduction alone does not eradicate *H. pylori*. Three- or four-drug therapy, including bismuth or (most often) proton pump inhibitor, combined with two antibiotics effective against *H. pylori*, will be necessary to eradicate the organism. Longer duration of therapy (i.e., 14 days) leads to a greater healing rate. This regimen will eradicate *H. pylori* in more than 90% of patients. Patients whose *H. pylori* has been eradicated have only approximately 5% chance of ulcer recurrence (compared to 60 to 70% of patients not treated for *H. pylori*). Generally, follow-up tests to prove *H. pylori* eradication are not recommended in the usual patient who becomes asymptomatic. If the peptic ulcer should recur (again, this happens infrequently), either direct testing of a biopsy specimen or a test for urease activity in the stomach (i.e., the C13 breath test) is necessary, as the serological studies remain positive for many years.

241. The answer is c. *(Braunwald, 15/e, pp 255–259.)* The first step in evaluating this patient with asymptomatic jaundice is to determine whether the increased bilirubin, as evidenced by scleral icterus, is conjugated or unconjugated hyperbilirubinemia. Patients with unconjugated hyperbilirubinemia do not have bilirubin in their urine because unconjugated bilirubin (bound to albumin) is not excreted in the urine; these patients usually have either hemolysis or an enzyme deficiency in the pathway for excretion of bilirubin. Conjugated hyperbilirubinemia suggests liver dysfunction and requires further assessment.

242. The answer is a. *(Braunwald, 15/e, pp 1784–1787.)* The patient has a conjugated hyperbilirubinemia with a cholestatic pattern of liver function tests. Normal transaminases rule out disease-causing hepatocellular damage (such as viral or alcoholic hepatitis). Instead, a disease of bile ducts or a cause of impaired bile excretion should be considered. Ultrasound or CT scan will evaluate the patient for biliary or pancreatic cancer or stone disease versus intrahepatic cholestasis.

243. The answer is a. *(Braunwald, 15/e, pp 260–262, 1762.)* Paracentesis is required to evaluate new-onset ascites. While cirrhosis and portal hypertension are most likely in this patient, complicating diseases such as tuberculous peritonitis and hepatoma are ruled out by analysis of ascitic fluid. An ultrasound or CT scan can be used to demonstrate ascitic fluid in equivocal cases.

244. The answer is a. *(Braunwald, 15/e, pp 260–262.)* A serum albumin minus ascitic fluid albumin greater than 1.1 suggests portal hypertension alone as a cause for ascites. Tuberculosis, pancreatitis, and malignancy would cause inflammation and increased capillary permeability, causing protein to leak into the ascitic fluid. This would result in a gradient between the serum and ascitic fluid of less than 1.1.

245. The answer is d. (*Braunwald, 15/e, pp 1764–1766.*) Hepatic encephalopathy presents as a change of consciousness, behavior, and neuromuscular function associated with liver disease. Hyperreflexia and asterixis (flapping tremor) are clinical manifestations of the disease process that result from toxins in the systemic circulation as a result of impaired hepatic clearance. Fever, gastrointestinal bleeding, and sedation are all potential precipitating factors in a patient with liver disease. Meningitis, subdural hematoma, and postictal state all occur in the alcoholic patient as well, and these may need to be distinguished from encephalopathy by additional tests such as lumbar puncture, CT scan, and EEG.

246. The answer is b. (*Braunwald, 15/e, pp 578–579, 1633–1634.*) The most likely diagnosis in this patient is esophageal carcinoma. Dysphagia is progressive, first for solids and then liquids. There is blood in the stool and a history of weight loss. Alcohol use and cigarette smoking are risk factors. Prognosis is not good, as once there is trouble swallowing, there is significant esophageal narrowing and the disease is usually incurable. A barium contrast study should demonstrate an esophageal carcinoma with marked narrowing and an irregular, ragged mucosal pattern. Formerly squamous cell carcinoma accounted for 90% of esophageal cancer, but its incidence is decreasing. Now more than 50% are adenocarcinomas, most often associated with Barrett's esophagus. Achalasia should not cause guaiac-positive stools or progressive symptoms.

247. The answer is a. (*Braunwald, 15/e, pp 1645–1647.*) In the absence of alarm symptoms (such as dysphagia, odynophagia, weight loss, or gastrointestinal bleeding), a therapeutic trial of acid reduction therapy is reasonable. Mild to moderate GERD symptoms often respond to H_2 blockers. More severe disease including erosive esophagitis usually requires proton pump inhibitor therapy for 8 weeks before healing. If the patient has recurrent symptoms or has had symptomatic GERD for over 5 years, endoscopy may be indicated to rule out Barrett's esophagus (gastric metaplasia of the lower esophagus). Barrett's esophagus is a premalignant condition, and most patients receive surveillance EGD every 2 to 3 years, although evidence of mortality benefit from this approach is not available. In the absence of alarm symptoms, a therapeutic trial is generally favored over the more expensive invasive approach.

248. The answer is c. *(Braunwald, 15/e, pp 579–581, 1665–1666, 1673–1675.)* The patient's history suggests malabsorption. Weight loss despite increased appetite goes with either a hypermetabolic state (such as hyperthyroidism) or nutrient malabsorption. The gastrointestinal symptoms support the diagnosis of malabsorption. Patients may notice greasy, malodorous stools, increase in stool frequency, stools that are tenacious and difficult to flush, as well as changes in bowel habits according to the fat content of the diet. In the United States, celiac sprue (gluten-sensitive enteropathy) and chronic pancreatic insufficiency are the commonest causes of malabsorption. The histological pattern in option c goes with sprue. IgA antiendomysial antibodies and antibodies against tissue glutaminase provide supporting evidence. Signet ring cells are seen with gastric cancer. This lesion can cause weight loss through anorexia or early satiety but would not cause malabsorption. The changes in option b go with ulcerative colitis; since this disease affects only the colon, small bowel absorption would not be affected. *Helicobacter pylori* is not associated with malabsorption.

249. The answer is b. *(Braunwald, 15/e, pp 1728–1734.)* The current hepatitis B vaccine is genetically engineered to consist of hepatitis B surface antigen particles. Therefore, only antibody to surface antigen will be detected after vaccination. Since the patient has had no exposure to hepatitis B, she should be surface antigen–negative; surface antigen positivity means active disease, either acute or chronic. Patients who have recovered from hepatitis B have antibodies both to HBS and HBC.

250–252. The answers are 250-a, 251-c, 252-b. *(Braunwald, 15/e, pp 255–259, 1785–1787.)* Primary biliary cirrhosis usually occurs in women between the ages of 35 and 60. The earliest symptom is pruritus, often accompanied by fatigue. Serum alkaline phosphatase is elevated two- to fivefold, and a positive antimitochondrial antibody test greater than 1:40 is both sensitive and specific. Diverticulitis predisposes to liver abscess, particularly in the elderly patient. Liver abscess should be suspected in any patient with a history of abdominal infection who develops jaundice and right upper quadrant pain. Obstructive jaundice that occurs in the setting of ulcerative colitis might be caused by gallstones or sclerosing cholangitis. Sclerosing cholangitis is a disorder characterized by a progressive inflammatory process of bile ducts. The diagnosis is usually made by demonstrating thickened ducts with narrow beaded lumina on cholangiography.

253. The answer is d. (*Braunwald, 15/e, pp 1661–1663.*) A young man with recurrent ulcer disease unresponsive to therapy should be evaluated for Zollinger-Ellison syndrome—gastrin-containing tumors that are usually in the pancreas. The patient's serum gastrin level is elevated, but not diagnostic for gastrinoma (>1000 pg/mL). A secretin injection induces marked increases in gastrin levels in all patients with gastrinoma. Once the diagnosis is made, CT scan or endoscopic ultrasound may help localize the tumor. Since these lesions arise from endocrine cells, they do not communicate with the pancreatic duct; ERCP would therefore not be helpful.

254. The answer is d. (*Braunwald, 15/e, pp 2257–2261.*) Hemochromatosis is a disorder of iron storage that results in deposition of iron in parenchymal cells. The liver is usually enlarged, and excessive skin pigmentation is present in 90% of symptomatic patients at the time of diagnosis. Diabetes occurs secondary to direct damage of the pancreas by iron deposition. Arthropathy develops in 25 to 50% of cases. Other diagnoses listed could not explain all the manifestations of this patient's disease process. Addison's disease can cause weight loss and hyperpigmentation but does not affect the liver or joints; it is associated with hypoglycemia rather than diabetes mellitus.

255–257. The answers are 255-a, 256-b, 257-c. (*Braunwald, 15/e, pp 255–259.*) The young African American male with mild jaundice has unconjugated hyperbilirubinemia and an anemia. This may be secondary to G6PD deficiency and an offending antibiotic (sulfonamide or trimethoprim-sulfamethoxazole). These patients are unable to maintain an adequate level of reduced glutathione in their red blood cells when an antibiotic or other toxin causes oxidative stress to the red cells. The 60-year-old male with jaundice has an obstructive process, as his pale stools suggest the lack of bilirubin in the stool. A high alkaline phosphatase also indicates that there is an obstructive jaundice. Pancreatic carcinoma would be the most likely cause of obstructive jaundice in this patient. The young woman's case is most consistent with acute hepatitis—very elevated hepatocellular enzymes and conjugated hyperbilirubinemia. Tenderness of the liver on palpation is common in acute hepatitis.

258. The answer is a. *(Braunwald, 15/e, pp 1692–1694.)* This patient meets the Rome criteria for irritable bowel syndrome. The major criterion is abdominal pain relieved with defecation and associated with change in stool frequency or consistency. In addition, these patients often complain of difficult stool passage, a feeling of incomplete evacuation, and mucus in the stool. In this young patient with long-standing symptoms and no evidence of organic disease on physical and laboratory studies, no further evaluation is necessary. Irritable bowel syndrome is a motility disorder associated with altered sensitivity to abdominal pain and distention. It is the commonest cause of chronic GI symptoms and is three times more common in women than in men. Associated lactose intolerance may cause similar symptoms and should be considered in all cases. Patients older than 40 years with new symptoms, weight loss, or positive family history of colon cancer should have further workup, usually with colonoscopy.

259. The answer is a. *(Braunwald, 15/e, pp 1799–1803.)* Chronic pancreatitis is due to pancreatic damage from recurrent attacks of acute pancreatitis. The classic triad is abdominal pain, malabsorption, and diabetes mellitus. Twenty-five percent of cases are idiopathic. Vitamins D and K are absorbed intact from the intestine without digestion by lipase and are therefore absorbed normally in pancreatic insufficiency. Forty percent of patients, however, develop B_{12} deficiency. Treatment of the malabsorption with pancreatic enzyme replacement will lead to weight gain, but the pain can be difficult to treat. Courvoisier's sign is a palpable, nontender gallbladder in a jaundiced patient. This finding suggests the presence of a malignancy, especially pancreatic cancer. Chronic pancreatitis per se does not produce guaiac-positive stools.

260. The answer is a. *(Braunwald, 15/e, pp 923–924.)* *C. difficile* is an important cause of diarrhea in patients who receive antibiotic therapy. *C. difficile* proliferates in the gastrointestinal tract when the normal enteric flora are altered by antibiotics. Commonly implicated antibiotics include ampicillin, penicillin, clindamycin, cephalosporins, and trimethoprim-sulfamethoxazole. The diarrhea is usually mild to moderate, but can occasionally be profound. Other clinical findings include pyrexia, abdominal pain, abdominal tenderness, leukocytosis, and serum electrolyte abnormalities. The diagnosis is made by demonstration at sigmoidoscopy of yellowish plaques (pseudomembranes) that cover the colonic mucosa or by detection of *C. difficile* toxin in the stool. The pseudomembranes consist of a tenacious fibrinopurulent mucosal exudate that contains extruded leukocytes, mucin, and sloughed mucosa. Isolation of *C. difficile* from stool cultures is not very specific because of asymptomatic carriage, particularly in infants. Serological tests are not clinically useful for diagnosing this infection. Pseudomembranous colitis demands discontinuation of the offending antibiotic. Antibiotic therapy for moderate or severe disease includes oral vancomycin or metronidazole. Cholestyramine and colestipol are also used therapeutically to bind the diarrheogenic toxin.

261–264. The answers are 261-a, 262-c, 263-b, 264-e. *(Braunwald, 15/e, pp 252–254.)* Nonsteroidal anti-inflammatory drugs, even over-the-counter brands, are common causes of GI bleeding. Often preceding symptoms are mild before the bleeding occurs. Cotreatment with misoprostol decreases GI bleeding but is quite expensive. Selective COX-2 inhibitors decrease the incidence of important GI bleeding and are preferred in the elderly.

Mallory-Weiss tears are linear mucosal tears at the gastroesophageal junction and cause painless GI bleeding. Although this patient has the classic history, half of all patients with Mallory-Weiss tears will notice blood with the initial vomitus. In this patient, endoscopy will be necessary to exclude bleeding varices, but the absence of clinical features of portal hypertension make this diagnosis less likely.

The erosion of the proximal end of a woven aortic graft into the distal duodenum or proximal jejunum can occur many years after the initial surgery. Often the patient will have a smaller herald bleed which is followed by catastrophic bleeding. A high index of suspicion is necessary as surgery can be lifesaving.

Patients with HHT usually have low-grade GI blood loss without obvious hematemesis; frequent nosebleeds may occur. The physical finding of small matlike telangiectasias of the mouth, lips, and fingertips points to this autosomal dominant disease and may prevent unnecessary endoscopy.

265–268. The answers are 265-a, 266-b, 267-a, 268-c. *(Braunwald, 15/e, pp 1679–1692.)* Ulcerative colitis may present with the acute or subacute onset of bloody diarrhea. Severe cases can cause toxic megacolon, a medical emergency. Colonic involvement starts in the rectum and proceeds toward the cecum in a continuous fashion. The biopsy findings, although characteristic, are not diagnostic, as infectious agents can cause the same changes. Exposure history and stool cultures will help make this distinction.

Crohn's disease can affect the entire GI tract from mouth to anus. Right lower quadrant pain, tenderness, and an inflammatory mass would suggest involvement of the terminal ileum. As opposed to ulcerative colitis (which is a mucosal disease), full-thickness involvement of the gut wall can lead to fistula and abscess formation. Skip lesions (i.e., segmental involvement) can also help distinguish Crohn's disease from UC; granuloma formation on biopsies would also support the diagnosis of Crohn's.

Although thought of as a disease of young adults, ulcerative colitis has a second peak of incidence in the 60- to 80-year age group and should be considered in the differential diagnosis of diarrhea at any age. Ischemic colitis also occurs in this age group. The ischemia is usually confined to the mucosa, so perforation is unusual. Pain is a prominent complaint and may mimic acute diverticulitis. The finding of segmental inflammation in watershed areas in the vascular distribution of the colon is characteristic. Most patients improve without surgical intervention.

269–272. The answers are 269-d, 270-c, 271-a, 272-b. *(Braunwald, 15/e, pp 241–243, 834–839.)* Giardiasis causes a subacute or chronic diarrhea with features of malabsorption. The protozoa plaster themselves to the small bowel mucosa and prevent intestinal absorption. Since the organisms are not invasive, white cells and RBCs are not seen in the stool. Travel history may suggest the diagnosis, but many cases are acquired from substandard drinking water supplies. A sensitive stool antigen test is now available.

Amebic dysentery, although rare in the U.S., is still common in developing nations. Cecal involvement is common, and extraintestinal manifestations (especially liver abscess) are often seen. A sensitive serological test is now available. Treatment is with high-dose metronidazole (750 mg TID for 5 to 10 days), although nonabsorbable agents may be used if extraintestinal disease is not present.

Foodborne illness (food poisoning) is a very common cause of acute GI symptoms. The short incubation period (indicating a preformed toxin rather than bacterial proliferation in the body) as well as the prominent upper GI symptoms are characteristic of staphylococcal food poisoning. *Salmonella* food poisoning is also common, but has a longer incubation period, usually causes diarrhea, and may be associated with fever and guaiac-positive stools indicating tissue invasion. Numerous other bacterial agents can cause acute symptoms.

Shigella often causes severe diarrhea with high fever, leukocytosis, and clinical toxicity. Distal colon involvement can cause tenesmus. Only a few hundred organisms can cause clinical infection, so point source outbreaks are frequent.

Nephrology

Questions

DIRECTIONS: Each item below contains a question or incomplete statement followed by suggested responses. Select the **one best** response to each question.

Items 273–276

273. A 76-year-old male presents to the emergency room. He had influenza and now presents with diffuse muscle pain and weakness. His past medical history is remarkable for osteoarthritis, for which he takes ibuprofen. Physical examination reveals a blood pressure of 130/90 with no orthostatic change. The only other finding is diffuse muscle tenderness. Laboratory data includes:

BUN: 30 mg/dL
Creatinine: 6 mg/dL
K: 6.0 meq/L
Uric acid: 18 mg/dL
Ca: 6.5 mg/dL
PO_4: 7.5 mg/dL
CPK: 28,000 IU/L
Urine output: 40 mL/h

Which is the most likely diagnosis?

a. Nonsteroidal anti-inflammatory drug–induced acute renal failure (ARF)
b. Volume depletion
c. Rhabdomyolysis-induced ARF
d. Urinary tract obstruction

274. Which diagnostic test is most useful for this patient?

a. Urine sodium
b. Urinalysis
c. Renal ultrasound
d. Urine uric acid–urine creatinine ratio

275. For this patient, which of the following is the initial therapy for rhabdomyolysis-induced ARF?

a. Mannitol
b. Dopamine
c. Natriuretic peptide
d. Alkaline diuresis

276. For this patient, which of the following would be a specific indication to start dialysis?

a. BUN rises to >90 mg/dL
b. Urine output falls to <10 mL/h
c. Pericardial friction rub develops
d. Hematocrit falls to <30%

277. A 68-year-old female with stable coronary artery disease undergoes angiography of the right lower extremity for peripheral vascular disease. The patient is on warfarin for recurrent deep vein thrombosis, aspirin, lisinopril, metoprolol, and atorvastatin. Preangiography, she received a course of dicloxacillin for cellulitis 1 week ago. Three weeks after angiography the patient is evaluated for general malaise. Physical examination reveals a petechial rash and livedo reticularis on both lower extremities. Laboratory evaluation reveals that her creatinine has risen from 1.5 to 3.7 mg/dL. Other laboratory abnormalities include an ESR of 96 mm/h, leukocytosis, eosinophiluria, and a reduced third component of complement (C_3). Urine sodium is 40 meq/L. Urinalysis reveals 1+ protein, 10 to 20 WBC/HPF, and 5 to 10 RBC/HPF with no casts. What is the most likely diagnosis?

a. Prerenal azotemia
b. Radiocontrast-induced acute renal failure
c. Drug-induced acute interstitial nephritis
d. Atheroembolic renal failure

278. A 46-year-old male with HIV and severe penicillin allergy receiving zidovudine, indinavir, and stavudine presents with fever, nonproductive cough, and severe hypoxia. Chest x-ray reveals diffuse increased interstitial markings and a possible lobar consolidation in the left lower lobe. After appropriate evaluation, the patient receives levofloxacin, trimethoprim-sulfamethoxazole, and acyclovir. Initial serum creatinine is 1.6 mg/dL. On day 4, it has risen to 3.8 mg/dL and a normal serum potassium has risen to 7.1 mg/dL. Urinalysis reveals no casts, 10 to 20 WBC/HPF, and rare RBCs. Which drug is the most likely cause of renal failure?

a. Levofloxacin
b. Trimethoprim-sulfamethoxazole
c. Acyclovir
d. Indinavir

Items 279–280

279. A 30-year-old male is brought to the emergency room from prison, where he works in the paint shop. He has no past medical history. CT scan of the head is normal. Urine toxicology screen is negative. Ethanol and acetaminophen are not detectable. Laboratory data is as follows:

Na: 138 meq/L
K: 4.2 meq/L
HCO_3: 5 meq/L
Cl: 104 meq/L
Creatinine: 1.0 mg/dL
BUN: 14 mg/dL
Ca: 10 mg/dL
Arterial blood gas on room air: Po_2 96, Pco_2 20, pH 7.02
Blood glucose: 90 mg/dL
Urinalysis: normal, without blood, protein, or crystals
Physical examination: blood pressure 100/60, with no orthostatic change
Neurological examination: barely arousable, no focal abnormalities, responds
    to deep pain

What is the acid-base disorder?

a. Non-anion-gap metabolic acidosis
b. Respiratory acidosis
c. Anion-gap metabolic acidosis
d. Anion-gap metabolic acidosis plus respiratory alkalosis

280. In this patient, which test will provide the key to correct diagnosis?

a. Serum ketones
b. Serum lactate
c. Salicylate level
d. Measured plasma osmolality

Items 281–282

281. A 70-year-old male is found lethargic at home with a blood pressure of 98/60 and a temperature of 98.6°F. In the emergency room, the following laboratory studies are obtained:

Na: 138 meq/L
K: 2.8 meq/L
HCO_3: 10 meq/L
Cl: 117 meq/L
BUN: 20 mg/dL
Creatinine: 1.0 mg/dL
Arterial blood gases: Po_2 80, Pco_2 25, pH 7.29
Urine pH: 4.5

What is the acid-base disorder?

a. Non-anion-gap metabolic acidosis
b. Respiratory acidosis
c. Anion-gap metabolic acidosis
d. Non-anion-gap metabolic acidosis and respiratory alkalosis

282. The most likely cause of the patient's disorder is

a. GI loss due to diarrhea
b. Proximal renal tubular acidosis
c. Distal renal tubular acidosis
d. Disorder of the renin-angiotensin-aldosterone system

Items 283–284

283. A 68-year-old female is found at home hypotensive (blood pressure 80/60) and confused. She has the following laboratory results in the emergency room:

Na: 130 meq/L
K: 2.6 meq/L
Cl: 70 meq/L
HCO_3: 50 meq/L
BUN: 40 mg/dL
Creatinine: 1.7 mg/dL
Arterial blood gases: PO_2 62, PCO_2 47, pH 7.63

Which acid-base disorder is present?

a. Metabolic alkalosis
b. Respiratory acidosis
c. Metabolic alkalosis plus respiratory acidosis
d. Respiratory alkalosis

284. Which of the following laboratory tests is most useful in determining the etiology of the acid-base disorder of this patient?

a. Urine sodium
b. Urine chloride
c. Urine pH
d. Urine potassium

285. A 43-year-old female presents with hypertension, edema, hyperlipidemia, and a deep venous thrombosis in her left leg. Which of the following is not necessary to diagnose the nephrotic syndrome?

a. Edema
b. Hypertension
c. 24-h urine albumin ≥3 g
d. Hyperlipidemia

DIRECTIONS: Each group of questions below consists of lettered options followed by a set of numbered items. For each numbered item, select the **one** lettered option with which it is **most** closely associated. Each lettered option may be used once, more than once, or not at all.

Items 286–289

Match the clinical and microscopic presentation with the correct primary glomerular disease.

a. Minimal change disease
b. Focal segmental sclerosis
c. Membranous nephropathy
d. Membranoproliferative glomerulonephritis

286. Hypertension, nephrotic syndrome, renal insufficiency, microhematuria, sclerotic changes in juxtamedullary nephrons **(CHOOSE 1 DISEASE)**

287. Mild hypertension, nephrotic syndrome, microhematuria, venous thromboses (especially renal vein thrombosis), thickened glomerular basement membrane with immunoglobulin deposition **(CHOOSE 1 DISEASE)**

288. Normal blood pressure, anasarca, severe nephrotic syndrome, normal light microscopy, fusion of foot processes on electron microscopy **(CHOOSE 1 DISEASE)**

289. Hypertension, nephrotic syndrome, mild renal insufficiency, RBC casts in urine, depressed third component of complement (C_3), dense deposits on electron microscopy **(CHOOSE 1 DISEASE)**

Items 290–291

290. A 63-year-old male alcoholic with a 50-pack-year history of smoking presents to the emergency room with fatigue and confusion. Physical examination reveals a blood pressure of 110/70 with no orthostatic change. Heart, lung, and abdominal examination are normal and there is no pedal edema. Laboratory data is as follows:

Na: 110 meq/L
K: 3.7 meq/L
Cl: 82 meq/L
HCO_3: 20 meq/L
Glucose: 100 mg/dL
BUN: 5 mg/dL
Creatinine: 0.7 mg/dL
Urinalysis: normal

The most likely diagnosis is

a. Volume depletion
b. Inappropriate secretion of antidiuretic hormone
c. Polydipsia
d. Cirrhosis

291. Which is the most useful first step in the assessment of hyponatremia in this patient?

a. Plasma arginine vasopressin
b. Urine sodium
c. Urine osmolality
d. Physical examination

292. A patient with a serum sodium of 110 meq/L suffers grand mal seizures. CT scan of the head and lumbar puncture are normal. What is the immediate treatment of the hyponatremia?

a. Normal saline at 250 mL/h
b. 750 mL oral fluid restriction
c. 3% saline at 30 to 40 mL/h plus furosemide
d. Demeclocycline

Items 293–295

293. A 65-year-old diabetic with a creatinine of 1.6 was started on an angiotensin converting enzyme inhibitor for hypertension and presents to the emergency room with weakness. His other medications include a statin for hypercholesterolemia, a beta blocker and spironolactone for congestive heart failure, insulin for diabetes, and aspirin. Laboratory examinations include:

K: 7.2 meq/L
Creatinine: 1.8
Glucose: 400 mg/dL
CPK: 400 IU/L

Which is the most important cause of hyperkalemia in this patient?

a. Worsening renal function
b. Uncontrolled diabetes
c. Statin-induced rhabdomyolysis
d. Drug-induced defects in the renin-angiotensin-aldosterone system

294. Which of the following is the most important factor in determining the initial treatment of hyperkalemia in this patient?

a. The magnitude of the hyperkalemia
b. The presence of renal failure
c. The presence of ECG changes consisting of a widened QRS
d. Severity of weakness

295. If this patient has a widened QRS on ECG, the first drug given is

a. Intravenous sodium bicarbonate
b. Intravenous calcium gluconate
c. Intravenous insulin
d. Polystyrene sulfonate (Kayexalate)

Items 296–299

Match the presentation with the systemic vasculitis.

a. Macroscopic polyarteritis nodosa
b. Wegener's granulomatosis
c. Essential mixed cryoglobulinemia
d. Systemic lupus erythematosus

296. An elderly male presenting with severe hypertension, abdominal pain, livedo reticularis, and mononeuritis multiplex **(CHOOSE 1 VASCULITIS)**

297. A Hispanic female, age 26, presenting with a malar rash, arthralgias of the hands, and edema **(CHOOSE 1 VASCULITIS)**

298. An older male presenting with sinopulmonary disease and rapidly progressive renal failure **(CHOOSE 1 VASCULITIS)**

299. A 35-year-old male with a history of intravenous drug abuse presenting with a purpuric rash on his legs, hypertension, and hematuria **(CHOOSE 1 VASCULITIS)**

300. You are designing a dialysis unit with dietitians, nurses, and pharmacologists to provide the best possible care. Patients suffering from which of the following conditions will make up your largest population?
a. Chronic glomerulonephritis
b. Hypertension
c. Diabetes mellitus
d. Obstructive uropathy

301. A 25-year-old female with diabetes mellitus presents with hypertension. The ideal target BP for pharmacologic control of hypertension is
a. ≤150/95
b. ≤135/85
c. ≤140/90
d. ≤125/75

302. A diabetic male presents with hypertension and 24-h urine showing 200 mg of albumin. In a diabetic patient with microalbuminuria, the appropriate drug for treatment of hypertension to prevent progression of renal failure is
a. Beta blocker
b. Thiazide diuretic
c. Angiotensin converting enzyme inhibitor
d. Short-acting dihydropyridine calcium channel blocker for precise control (nifedipine)

Items 303–306

Match the type of stone with the clinical situation in which it occurs.

a. Calcium oxalate
b. Cystine
c. Struvite
d. Uric acid

303. Low urine pH **(CHOOSE 1 STONE TYPE)**

304. Chronically infected urine **(CHOOSE 1 STONE TYPE)**

305. Hexagonal urinary crystals; intractable stone disease beginning in childhood **(CHOOSE 1 STONE TYPE)**

306. Regional enteritis **(CHOOSE 1 STONE TYPE)**

307. A 29-year-old male with HIV, on indinavir, zidovudine, and stavudine, presents with severe edema and a serum creatinine of 2.0 mg/dL. He has had bone pain for 5 years and takes large amounts of acetominophen with codeine, aspirin, and ibuprofen. He is on prophylactic trimethoprim sulfamethoxazole. Blood pressure is 170/110; urinalysis shows 4+ protein, 5 to 10 RBC, 0 WBC; 24-h urine protein is 6.2 g. What is the most likely cause of his renal disease?

a. Indinavir toxicity
b. Analgesic nephropathy
c. Trimethoprim sulfamethoxazole–induced interstitial nephritis
d. Focal sclerosis

Nephrology

Answers

273. The answer is c. *(Braunwald, 15/e, pp 1508–1510.)* Rhabdomyolysis-induced ARF may follow influenza. It is characterized by a creatinine disproportionately elevated compared to BUN (usual BUN-creatinine ratio ~ 10), hyperkalemia, hyperphosphatemia, and hyperuricemia, all due to release of intracellular muscle products. The high phosphorus causes hypocalcemia. All nonsteroidal agents may cause decreased renal function. Usually this is due to decreased blood flow—less commonly, to drug-induced nephritis. The laboratory abnormalities discussed are not seen in either situation. However, stopping the ibuprofen in this patient would be prudent. The absence of orthostatic hypotension makes the diagnosis of volume depletion very unlikely. Nothing on history, physical examination, or electrolyte abnormalities suggests obstruction. However, in a 76-year-old man, considering occult obstruction is always appropriate.

274. The answer is b. *(Braunwald, 15/e, pp 1546–1547.)* Urinalysis showing muddy brown granular casts is diagnostic of acute tubular necrosis and consistent with rhabdomyolysis-induced ARF. In oliguric (<20 mL urine per hour) ARF, a urine sodium less than 10 meq/L suggests prerenal azotemia; a value greater than 20 meq/L suggests acute tubular necrosis. Urine sodium is not useful in nonoliguric ARF (greater than 20 mL urine per hour). Obstructive uropathy is unlikely with the multiple electrolyte disorders in this patient. However, renal ultrasound is an appropriate test in a 76-year-old male to be sure occult obstruction is not contributing to renal failure. Despite the high serum uric acid, acute urate nephropathy does not occur with rhabdomyolysis. Acute urate nephropathy may occur with chemotherapy of aggressive tumors (e.g., Burkitt's lymphoma) and is characterized by a urine uric acid–creatinine ratio greater than 1.

275. The answer is d. *(Braunwald, 15/e, pp 1548–1549.)* Rhabdomyolysis-induced ARF is partly due to tubular obstruction by myoglobin and partly due to nephrotoxicity of myoglobin. Diuresis may relieve obstruction, and alkalization of the urine with bicarbonate may decrease nephrotoxicity of myoglobin. Frequently used in the past, mannitol no longer has a role in

ARF. Low-dose dopamine may increase renal blood flow, but does not improve ARF. Natriuretic peptide has many theoretical hemodynamic effects, but has not been proved to improve ARF.

276. The answer is c. (*Braunwald, 15/e, p 1546.*) Pericarditis in renal failure (acute or chronic) is an indication to initiate hemodialysis, because untreated uremic pericarditis may progress to pericardial tamponade. Other indications include encephalopathy, volume overload, and intractable hyperkalemia. There is no absolute number for BUN to initiate dialysis. No degree of oliguria is a specific indication for dialysis, although this situation must be closely watched for volume overload. Bone marrow depression, mainly due to reduced erythropoetin combined with mildly reduced red cell half-life, causes hematocrit to fall almost universally in renal failure (acute and chronic). This does not determine need for dialysis.

277. The answer is d. (*Braunwald, 15/e, p 1544.*) Atheroembolic renal failure is a poorly understood syndrome of subacute renal failure in patients with severe vascular disease who undergo angiography. For unknown reasons, warfarin appears to be a risk factor. Clinical features include the dermatologic findings in this patient, refractile plaques in the retinal arteries (Hollenhorst plaques), and digital cyanosis. Although atheroembolic renal failure was once felt to lead inevitably to end-stage renal disease, it is now recognized that a significant percentage of patients have some recovery of renal function. Volume depletion is not associated with the physical findings and diverse laboratory abnormalities seen in this patient. A urine sodium less than 10 meq/L would be expected if the patient is oliguric. Radiocontrast-induced acute renal failure occurs immediately after contrast studies and lacks the physical findings and diverse laboratory abnormalities seen in this patient. Dicloxacillin may cause drug-induced acute interstitial nephritis, which is characterized by fever, diffuse erythematous rash, white blood cell casts in the urine, and eosinophiluria. As this entity is treatable with corticosteroids, a renal biopsy would be indicated to exclude it.

278. The answer is b. (*Braunwald, 15/e, p 879.*) In the elderly or in patients with renal insufficiency, full doses of trimethoprim-sulfamethonazole frequently cause drug-induced interstitial nephritis and hyperkalemia (due to inhibition of the sodium-potassium transport system in the distal nephron). Levofloxacin is a very rare cause of renal dysfunction. In the setting of volume depletion, acyclovir may cause acute renal failure secondary to intratubular obstruction from crystal deposition. Crystals are absent from the urine in this case. Indinavir may crystallize and cause either nephrolithiasis or renal failure due to tubular obstruction.

279. The answer is c. *(Braunwald, 15/e, p 284.)* The pH is low, so the primary process is acidosis. The serum HCO_3 has decreased from 24 to 5 meq/L, so this is a metabolic acidosis. The PCO_2 is 20 mmHg, down from a normal 40 mmHg, a normal compensation (PCO_2 decreases by 1 to 1.5 mgHg for each 1-meq decrease in HCO_3). The normal anion gap (Na − [Cl + HCO_3]) is 8 to 12 meq/L; here it is 29 meq/L. Thus this is an anion-gap metabolic acidosis with appropriate respiratory compensation. A brief differential of anion-gap metabolic acidosis is as follows:

Diabetic ketoacidosis
Lactic acidosis
Alcoholic ketoacidosis
Toxic alcohol ingestion (methanol, ethylene glycol)
Salicylate intoxication
Renal failure

Non-anion-gap metabolic acidosis is excluded by the anion gap of 31. Respiratory acidosis is excluded by the low PCO_2. Anion-gap metabolic acidosis plus respiratory alkalosis is excluded because the PCO_2 of 20 mmHg is appropriate compensation, not true respiratory alkalosis.

280. The answer is d. *(Braunwald, 15/e, p 287.)* Plasma osmolality is calculated as follows: 2 × Na + BUN/2.8 + glucose/18 + blood ethanol/4.6 (denominators are a function of molecular weight). Here the calculated osmolality is 288 mosm/L (2 × 138 + 14/2.8 + 90/18 + 0/4.6). Assume a measured plasma osmolality of 320 mosm/L. The measured osmolality of 320 mosm/L minus the calculated osmolality of 288 mosm/L is 32 (nl less than 10), consistent with a large osmolar gap, due either to methanol or ethylene glycol. In this case, methanol, used in paint thinners, is likely. Ethylene glycol, used in antifreeze, is frequently associated with hypocalcemia, renal failure, and crystalluria. Serum ketones should be checked, but diabetic ketoacidosis is unlikely with a blood sugar of 90 mg/dL, and alcoholic ketoacidosis rarely, if ever, causes acidosis of this severity. Serum lactate should be checked, but in an afebrile patient with normal blood pressure lactic acidosis is unlikely to be the primary cause. Elevated salicylate level causes mixed metabolic acidosis–respiratory alkalosis with a near normal pH in the adult. In an infant, severe metabolic acidosis may occur.

281. The answer is a. (*Braunwald, 15/e, p 286.*) With a pH of 7.29, the primary process is acidosis. The HCO_3 is low (10 meq/L) and the anion gap is normal at 11 meq/L, and the PCO_2 of 29 mmHg is appropriate respiratory compensation. Thus this is a non-anion-gap metabolic acidosis with appropriate respiratory compensation. A brief differential diagnosis is as follows:

GI HCO_3 loss below the ligament of Treitz
Renal HCO_3 (proximal renal tubular acidosis, distal renal tubular acidosis)
Defects of the renin-angiotensin-aldosterone axis
Early chronic renal failure

Respiratory acidosis is not consistent with PCO_2 of 25 mmHg. Anion-gap metabolic acidosis is not consistent with a normal anion gap. Non-anion-gap metabolic acidosis and respiratory alkalosis are not present because the PCO_2 represents normal compensation for acute acidosis.

282. The answer is a. (*Braunwald, 15/e, pp 287–288.*) Non-anion-gap acidosis, hypokalemia, and low urine pH are all consistent with gastrointestinal loss due to diarrhea. Proximal renal tubular acidosis is a primary disorder found mainly in early childhood. It may be seen in unusual adult systemic diseases, but not as an acute acidosis. Urine pH is usually high. Distal renal tubular acidosis is excluded by a urine pH of less than 6. Disorders of the renin-angiotensin-aldosterone system are a common cause of hyperchloremic acidosis in older patients, but defects in aldosterone function invariably cause hyperkalemia, not hypokalemia.

283. The answer is a. (*Braunwald, 15/e, pp 288–289.*) The pH is high and the plasma HCO_3 is high, consistent with metabolic alkalosis. The respiratory compensation is limited by hypoxic drive. Usually when the PCO_2 rises to the high 40s or low 50s, hypoxic drive is stimulated to maintain a $PO_2 >$ 60 mgHg as in the present case. A brief differential diagnosis is as follows:

Low or normal blood pressure
    Upper GI loss above the ligament of Treitz
    Renal loss (e.g., due to diuretics)

Increased blood pressure
  Primary aldosteronism
  Cushing's disease or syndrome
  Any mineralocorticoid excess
Miscellaneous
  Bartter syndrome

Respiratory acidosis cannot be the primary abnormality with high pH. Metabolic alkalosis plus respiratory acidosis is excluded because the increased P_{CO_2} represents appropriate compensation, not a primary disorder. Respiratory alkalosis is impossible with high P_{CO_2}.

284. The answer is b. *(Braunwald, 15/e, p 289.)* This patient has low blood pressure and metabolic alkalosis. Therefore, her disorder is due either to GI loss (e.g., vomiting) or to renal loss (e.g., furosemide). Urine chloride will be low in the former and high in the latter (except if off diuretics for days). Urine sodium will not differentiate GI from renal losses and is likely to be surprisingly high in both. With a plasma HCO_3 of 50, obligatory renal loss of HCO_3 will occur, requiring cation loss (either sodium or potassium) to maintain electroneutrality. Urine HCO_3 loss will cause a high urine pH with a plasma HCO_3 of 50. Urine HCO_3 loss plus high levels of aldosterone due to volume depletion will cause urinary potassium loss despite hypokalemia.

285. The answer is b. *(Braunwald, 15/e, pp 1584–1585.)* While hypertension may occur in diseases causing the nephrotic syndrome, its presence is not necessary for the diagnosis of this syndrome. Renal loss and catabolism of albumin lead to hypoalbuminemia and edema. Increased hepatic synthesis of lipoproteins leads to markedly elevated lipid levels.

286–289. The answers are 286-b, 287-c, 288-a, 289-d. *(Braunwald, 15/e, pp 1585–1588.)* Minimal change disease is commonest in children; hypertension or renal failure is rare, and generally the condition is responsive to corticosteroid therapy. Focal segmental sclerosis is common in African Americans, frequently progresses to end-stage renal disease, and is relatively refractory to therapy. Membranous nephropathy is the commonest cause of idiopathic nephrotic syndrome in adults. One-third of cases improve spontaneously, one-third remain stable, and one-third progress to end-stage renal disease if untreated. The condition is fairly responsive to corticosteroid and cytotoxic therapy. Membranoproliferative glomerulo-nephritis is the rarest cause of idiopathic nephrotic syndrome in adults. Depressed C_3 is due to an autoantibody that is not pathogenetic. Erratic clinical course and erratic response to therapy are typical.

290. The answer is b. (*Braunwald, 15/e, pp 274–275.*) Inappropriate secretion of antidiuretic hormone is a diagnosis of exclusion, but a chest x-ray might reveal a lung mass. This syndrome may be idiopathic, associated with certain pulmonary and intracranial pathologies, due to endocrine disorders (e.g., hypothyroidism), or drug-induced (e.g., many psychotropic agents). Significant volume depletion is excluded by the absence of orthostatic hypotension. As one can excrete 20% of the glomerular filtration rate, one would have to ingest more than 20 L/day to become hyponatremic. Cirrhosis is very unlikely in the absence of ascites and edema.

291. The answer is d. (*Braunwald, 15/e, pp 274–275.*) Physical examination is the most important first step. Hyponatremia tells us about the tonicity of plasma, not about total body sodium. Hyponatremic patients may have low total body sodium (e.g., volume depletion), which will cause orthostatic hypotension; high total body sodium (e.g., congestive heart failure, cirrhosis, nephrotic syndrome), which will cause edema; or normal body sodium (inappropriate antidiuretic hormone secretion) with neither of the above. Plasma arginine vasopressin will be high in all hyponatremic states except the rare case of polydipsia. Urine sodium can be high or low with volume depletion (diarrhea versus diuretics) and high or low with inappropriate antidiuretic hormone secretion (reflecting dietary intake). Urine osmolality is high in all these states due to high arginine vasopressin levels.

292. The answer is c. (*Braunwald, 15/e, p 276.*) Seizures due to severe hyponatremia are a medical emergency. Hypertonic saline at this slow rate plus furosemide to create an isotonic urine will correct the hyponatremia at ½ to 1 meq/h. Overly rapid correction can lead to irreversible central pontine myelinolysis. Depending on the urine osmolality, normal saline at 250 mL/h may fail to help and may potentially aggravate the situation. Oral fluid restriction to 750 mL is appropriate, but will not help acutely. Demeclocycline induces nephrogenic diabetes insipidus and may play a role in chronic therapy. Avoid it in the setting of liver disease, as death from liver failure has occurred.

293. The answer is d. *(Braunwald, 15/e, pp 281–282.)* The syndrome of hyporeninemic hypoaldosteronism occurs in older diabetics, particularly males with congestive heart failure. The syndrome often presents when aggravating drugs are added. Beta blockers impair renin secretion, converting enzyme inhibitors decrease aldosterone levels, and spironolactone competes for the aldosterone receptor. Combined with diabetes and mild renal insufficiency, the result may be significant hyperkalemia. The moderate increase in creatinine is unlikely to cause severe hyperkalemia. The hypertonicity due to hyperglycemia could aggravate hyperkalemia, but a blood glucose of 400 mg/dL should not cause severe hyperkalemia. Statin drugs may cause muscle injury and rhabdomyolysis, but a CPK of 400 IU/L is a modest elevation and would not cause severe hyperkalemia.

294. The answer is c. *(Braunwald, 15/e, p 282.)* Hyperkalemia induces a series of ECG changes progressing from peaked T waves to a widened QRS to asystole. The evidence of target organ effects (especially on the heart), not the degree of hyperkalemia, determines initial therapy. The presence or absence of renal failure, not the initial treatment, determines how potassium will ultimately be removed (polystyrene sulfonate, diuretics, or dialysis). Weakness due to hyperkalemia does not affect the respiratory muscle; since respiratory failure does not occur, weakness does not determine initial therapy.

295. The answer is b. *(Braunwald, 15/e, pp 282–283.)* Within 1 to 3 min, intravenous calcium gluconate begins to reverse the ECG effects of hyperkalemia by normalizing membrane excitability. Sodium bicarbonate may be helpful in shifting potassium into cells beginning in 15 to 30 min. Effects are not always predictable, and sodium load may aggravate congestive heart failure. Intravenous insulin is effective at shifting potassium into cells, but requires 15 to 30 min. Don't forget to give enough glucose to prevent hypoglycemia. Polystyrene sulfonate (Kayexalate) is a gastrointestinal cation exchange resin. It is useful for removing potassium, but has no role in acute therapy.

296–299. The answers are 296-a, 297-d, 298-b, 299-c. *(Braunwald, 15/e, pp 1576, 1922–1928, 1958–1963.)* Macroscopic polyarteritis nodosa is a vasculitis of medium-sized blood vessels that causes renal artery aneurysms (severe hypertension), abdominal aneurysms (abdominal pain), and vascular damage to skin and peripheral nerves. Patients are most commonly older males and anyone who is hepatitis B surface antigen positive. Small-vessel vasculitis is most common in older males with granulomatous inflammation of the upper respiratory tract and kidneys and is associated with a positive c-ANCA (antineutrophil cytoplasmic antibody) test. Associated with hepatitis C, essential mixed cryoglobulinemia most commonly affects the skin and kidneys. Treatment is aimed at the hepatitis with interferon and ribavirin. SLE has a predilection for young African American and Hispanic females and has protean manifestations, especially a malar rash, arthralgias of the hands, and renal involvement. It is associated with a positive ANA (rim pattern) and antibodies against double-stranded DNA.

300. The answer is c. *(Braunwald, 15/e, p 1551.)* Diabetes mellitus, by far the commonest cause of end-stage renal disease in the United States, is responsible for more than 40% of new dialysis cases each year. Chronic glomerulonephritis is a somewhat nonspecific diagnosis; this is the third commonest cause. Hypertension is the second leading cause of end-stage renal disease in the U.S., and disproportionately affects African Americans. All patients with renal failure should have obstruction ruled out early; this should not lead to end-stage renal disease.

301. The answer is b. *(Braunwald, 15/e, p 2125.)* The current target blood pressure for all patients with diabetes mellitus is ≤135/85. Blood pressure ≤150/95 is an outdated standard. Blood pressure ≤140/90 is the current definition of normal, above which some intervention (not necessarily pharmacologic) is indicated. Blood pressure ≤125/75 is the challenging goal in patients with diabetic nephropathy to limit progression of disease.

302. The answer is c. *(Braunwald, 15/e, p 2128.)* By a variety of mechanisms, angiotensin converting enzyme inhibitors help to preserve renal function in this situation. Two caveats: be sure to monitor serum potassium, and, in the older patient with potential renal vascular disease, monitor serum creatinine after initiation of therapy. Although many diabetic patients receive beta blockers due to coronary disease, these are not first-line drugs for preventing progression of renal failure. Caution is necessary in using beta blockers, as they may blunt the symptoms and physiologic response to hypoglycemia. Because of low cost and proven efficacy, thiazide diuretics remain a good choice for the general population, but do not have a specific effect on progression of renal disease. Short-acting dihydropyridine calcium channel blockers (nifedipine) may increase the incidence of stroke and myocardial infarction, and have no role in the treatment of hypertension.

303–306. The answers are 303-d, 304-c, 305-b, 306-a. *(Braunwald, 15/e, pp 1618, 1619.)* Uric acid stones are associated with low urine pH. Low urine pH (due to decreased NH_3 production by the kidney) is the commonest cause of radiolucent uric acid stones. Urate is underexcreted in an acid urine. Struvite stones are found in chronically infected urine. Especially with *Proteus* infections, urinary pH rises to 8, causing precipitation of $MgNH_4PO_4$ into staghorn calculi. Stones are opaque. Hexagonal urinary crystals are found in cystinuria, an uncommon hereditary disease that leads to urinary wasting of cystine, ornithine, lysine, and arginine (COLA). Cystine stones start early in life and if untreated progress to end-stage renal disease. Stones may be lucent or opaque. Regional enteritis of the small intestine leads to increased oxalate absorption and formation of calcium stones. Stones are radiopaque.

307. The answer is d. *(Braunwald, 15/e, p 1887.)* Although many glomerular lesions occur in association with HIV, focal sclerosis is by far the commonest etiology of this patient's syndrome. While focal sclerosis is more common in intravenous drug users than homosexuals, the lesion is different than so-called heroin nephropathy. Indinavir toxicity may cause tubular obstruction by crystals and is a cause of renal stones, but does not cause nephrotic syndrome. Analgesic nephropathy is a frequently unrecognized cause of occult renal failure; this entity requires at least 10 years of analgesic use and rarely causes significant proteinuria. Trimethoprim-sulfamethoxazole may cause acute interstitial nephritis, but there is no fever, rash, WBC casts, or eosinophils in the urinalysis.

Hematology and Oncology

Questions

DIRECTIONS: Each item below contains a question or incomplete statement followed by suggested responses. Select the **one best** response to each question.

308. A 55-year-old male is being evaluated for constipation. There is no history of prior gastrectomy or of upper GI symptoms. Hemoglobin is 10 g/dL, mean corpuscular volume (MCV) is 72 fL, serum iron is 4 μg/dL (normal is 50 to 150 μg/dL), iron-binding capacity is 450 μg/dL (normal is 250 to 370 μg/dL), saturation is 1% (normal is 20 to 45%), and ferritin is 10 μg/L (normal is 15 to 400 μg/L). The next step in the evaluation of this patient's anemia is

a. Red blood cell folate
b. Iron absorption studies
c. Colonoscopy
d. Bone marrow examinaton

309. A 50-year-old woman complains of pain and swelling in her proximal interphalangeal joints, both wrists, and both knees. She complains of morning stiffness. She had a hysterectomy 10 years ago. Physical exam shows swelling and thickening of the PIP joints. Hemoglobin is 10.3 g/dL, MCV is 80 fL, serum iron is 8 μmol/L, iron-binding capacity is 200 μg/dL (normal is 250 to 370 μg/dL), and saturation is 10%. The most likely explanation for this woman's anemia is

a. Occult blood loss
b. Vitamin deficiency
c. Anemia of chronic disease
d. Sideroblastic anemia

310. A 35-year-old female who is recovering from *Mycoplasma* pneumonia develops increasing weakness. Her Hgb is 9.0 g/dL and her MCV is 110. The best test to determine whether the patient has a hemolytic anemia is

a. Serum bilirubin
b. Reticulocyte count and blood smear
c. *Mycoplasma* antigen
d. Serum LDH

Items 311–313

311. A 70-year-old male complains of 2 months of low back pain and fatigue. He has developed fever with purulent sputum production. On physical exam, he has pain over several vertebrae and rales at the left base. Laboratory results are as follows:

Hemoglobin: 7 g/dL
MCV: 86 fL (normal 86 to 98)
WBC: 12,000/μL
BUN: 44 mg/dL
Creatinine: 3.2 mg/dL
Ca: 11.5 mg/dL
Chest x-ray: LLL infiltrate
Reticulocyte count: 1%

The most likely diagnosis is

a. Multiple myeloma
b. Lymphoma
c. Metastatic bronchogenic carcinoma
d. Primary hyperparathyroidism

312. The definitive diagnosis is best made by

a. 24-h urine protein
b. Greater than 10% plasma cells in bone marrow
c. Renal biopsy
d. Rouleaux formation on blood smear

313. Renal insufficiency may have developed in this patient secondary to

a. Obstruction of collecting tubules by Bence-Jones protein
b. Hypercalcemia
c. Amyloid deposition
d. Plasma cell infiltration of the kidney
e. All of the above

314. After undergoing surgical resection for carcinoma of the stomach, a 60-year-old male develops numbness in his feet. On exam, he has lost proprioception in the lower extremities and has a wide-based gait and positive Romberg sign. A peripheral blood smear shows macrocytosis and hypersegmented polymorphonuclear leukocytes. The neurologic dysfunction is secondary to a deficiency of which vitamin?

a. Folic acid
b. Thiamine
c. Vitamin K
d. Vitamin B_{12}

Items 315–316

315. A 60-year-old asymptomatic man is found to have a leukocytosis when a routine CBC is obtained. Physical exam shows no abnormalities. The spleen is of normal size. Lab data includes:

Hgb: 9 g/dL (normal 14 to 18)
Leukocytes: 40,000/µL (normal 4,300 to 10,800)

Peripheral blood smear shows a differential that includes 97% small lymphocytes. The most likely diagnosis is

a. Acute monocytic leukemia
b. Chronic myelogenous leukemia
c. Chronic lymphocytic leukemia
d. Tuberculosis

316. This patient will require chemotherapy

a. If the white blood cell count rises
b. If lymphadenopathy develops
c. To control anemia or thrombocytopenia
d. Only when acute lymphocytic leukemia develops

317. A 67-year-old male presents with hemoptysis 1 week in duration. He has smoked 1½ packs of cigarettes per day for 50 years and has been unable to quit smoking despite nicotine replacement therapy and bupropion. He has mild COPD for which he uses an ipratropium inhaler. Chest x-ray reveals a 3-cm perihilar mass. The most likely cause of this patient's hemoptysis is

a. Adenocarcinoma of the lung
b. Squamous cell carcinoma of the lung
c. Bronchoalveolar cell carcinoma
d. Bronchial adenoma

318. A 38-year-old female presents with recurrent sore throats. She is on no medications, does not use ethanol, and has no history of renal disease. Physical exam is normal. A CBC shows Hgb of 9.0 g/dL, MCV is 85 fL (normal), white blood cell count is 2,000/μL, and platelet count is 30,000/μL. The best approach to diagnosis is

a. Erythropoietin level
b. Serum B_{12}
c. Bone marrow biopsy
d. Liver spleen scan

Items 319–320

319. A 50-year-old female complains of vague abdominal pain, constipation, and a sense of fullness in the lower abdomen. On physical exam the abdomen is nontender, but there is shifting dullness to percussion. The next step in evaluation is

a. Abdominal ultrasound
b. Pelvic examination
c. CA 125 cancer antigen
d. Sigmoidoscopy

320. This patient was found to have a right adnexal mass on physical examination. Abdominal ultrasound confirms the finding. Abdominal paracentesis reveals malignant cells consistent with ovarian cancer. Risk factors for this malignancy include

a. Infertility
b. Oral contraceptives
c. Coitus early in life
d. Multiple sexual partners

Items 321–322

321. A 40-year-old male complains of hematuria and an aching pain in his flank. Laboratory data show normal BUN, creatinine, and electrolytes. Hemoglobin is elevated at 18 g/dL and serum calcium is 11 mg/dL. A solid renal mass is found by ultrasound. The most likely diagnosis is

a. Polycystic kidney disease
b. Renal carcinoma
c. Adrenal adenoma
d. Urolithiasis

322. The best choice for cure in this patient is

a. Nephrectomy
b. Radiation therapy
c. Interferon α
d. Interleukin 2

323. A 20-year-old male finds a mass in his scrotum. The first step in evaluating this mass is

a. Palpation and transillumination
b. HCG and α-fetoprotein
c. Scrotal ultrasonography
d. Evaluation for inguinal adenopathy

324. A 65-year-old man presents with painless hematuria. He has a 45-year history of tobacco use. He denies fever, chills, and dysuria. General physical exam is unremarkable. On rectal exam, the prostate is small, nonnodular, and nontender. A urinalysis shows 100 red blood cells per high-power field. No white cells or protein are present. Three months previously, the patient had an abdominal ultrasound for right upper quadrant pain; on review, both kidneys were normal. The most useful diagnostic test at this time is

a. Urine culture and sensitivity
b. PSA
c. Renal biopsy
d. Cystoscopy

Items 325–326

325. A patient complains of fatigue and night sweats associated with itching for 2 months. On physical exam, there is diffuse nontender lymphadenopathy, including small supraclavicular, epitrochlear, and scalene nodes. A chest x-ray shows hilar lymphadenopathy. The next step in evaluation is

a. Excisional lymph node biopsy
b. Monospot test
c. Toxoplasmosis IgG
d. Serum angiotensin converting enzyme level

326. The patient is found on biopsy to have mixed-cellularity Hodgkin's lymphoma. Liver function tests are normal, and the spleen is nonpalpable. The next step in evaluation is

a. CT scan of abdomen and pelvis
b. Liver biopsy
c. Staging laparotomy
d. Erythrocyte sedimentation rate

Items 327–328

327. A 62-year-old African American man presents with fatigue, decreased urine stream, and low back pain. The physical examination shows a hard, nodular left prostatic lobe and percussion tenderness in the lumbar vertebral bodies and left seventh rib. The next step in evaluation is

a. Bone scan ·
b. Biopsy of prostate
c. CT scan
d. Bone marrow biopsy

328. The patient is found to have adenocarcinoma of the prostate with bony metastases. Treatment of choice is

a. Observation
b. Radiation therapy
c. Estrogen therapy
d. Gonadotropin-releasing hormone (GnRH) analogue
e. Chemotherapy

Items 329–330

329. A 64-year-old male is hospitalized with a transient ischemic attack and is evaluated for carotid disease. Physical exam is normal. CBC on admission is normal. The patient is started on heparin. A repeat CBC 1 week later shows an Hgb of 14 g/dL (normal is 13 to 18 g/dL), WBC of 9,000/μL, and platelet count of 10,000/μL. You should

a. Obtain a bone marrow study
b. Obtain a liver-spleen scan
c. Suspect drug-induced thrombocytopenia
d. Begin corticosteroids for idiopathic thrombocytopenia purpura

330. The patient described develops thrombosis of the brachial artery. The next step in management is

a. Lupus anticoagulant
b. Antinuclear antibody
c. Lepirudin or danaparoid
d. Increased heparin dose

331. A patient with bacterial endocarditis develops thrombophlebitis while hospitalized. His course in the hospital is uncomplicated. On discharge he is treated with penicillin, rifampin, and warfarin. Therapeutic prothrombin levels are obtained on 15 mg/d of warfarin. After 2 weeks, the penicillin and rifampin are discontinued. You should now

a. Cautiously increase warfarin dosage
b. Continue warfarin at 15 mg/d for about 6 months
c. Reduce warfarin dosage
d. Stop warfarin therapy

332. A 65-year-old male with diabetes mellitus, bronzed skin, and cirrhosis of the liver is being treated for hemochromatosis previously confirmed by liver biopsy. The patient experiences increasing right upper quadrant pain, and his serum alkaline phosphatase is now elevated. There is a 15-lb weight loss. The next step in management is

a. Increase frequency of phlebotomy for worsening hemochromatosis
b. Obtain CT scan to rule out hepatoma
c. Obtain hepatitis B serology
d. Obtain antimitochondrial antibody to rule out primary biliary cirrhosis

333. A 40-year-old cigarette smoker is found on routine physical exam to have a 1-cm white patch on his oral mucosa that does not rub off. There are no other lesions in the mouth. The patient has no risk factors for HIV infection. The lesion is nontender. The next step in management is

a. Culture for *Candida albicans*
b. Follow lesion with annual physical exam
c. Refer to oral surgeon for biopsy of lesion
d. Reassure patient that this is a normal variant

DIRECTIONS: Each group of questions below consists of lettered options followed by a set of numbered items. For each numbered item, select the **one** lettered option with which it is **most** closely associated. Each lettered option may be used once, more than once, or not at all.

Items 334–338

Match the chemotherapeutic agent with the anticipated response.

a. Better than 50% chance that the lesion will be cured
b. Prolongation of survival
c. Palliation
d. Little or no response

334. A 25-year-old male with nonseminomatous testicular cancer and lung metastases **(CHOOSE 1 RESPONSE)**

335. Malignant melanoma with lung metastases **(CHOOSE 1 RESPONSE)**

336. Breast cancer with bone metastases **(CHOOSE 1 RESPONSE)**

337. Stage III B Hodgkin's disease **(CHOOSE 1 RESPONSE)**

338. Small cell carcinoma of the lung with liver and bone metastases **(CHOOSE 1 RESPONSE)**

339. A 20-year-old black male with sickle cell anemia (SS homozygote) has had several episodes of painful crises. The least likely physical finding in this patient is

a. Scleral icterus
b. Systolic murmur
c. Splenomegaly
d. Ankle ulcers

340. A 30-year-old black man plans a trip to India and is advised to take prophylaxis for malaria. Three days after beginning treatment, he develops dark urine, pallor, fatigue, and jaundice. Hematocrit is 30% (it had been 43%) and reticulocyte count is 7%. He stops taking the medication. Treatment should consist of

a. Splenectomy
b. Administration of methylene blue
c. Administration of vitamin E
d. Exchange transfusions
e. No additional treatment is required

Items 341–342

341. A 58-year-old Scandinavian male presents with shortness of breath and is found to have anemia. Peripheral blood smear shows macrocytosis and hypersegmented polyps. The patient also has postural hypotension. Skin shows both vitiligo and hyperpigmentation. Romberg sign is positive. Serum sodium is 120 meq/L (normal is 136 to 145 meq/L) and potassium is 5.2 meq/L (normal is 3.5 to 5.0 meq/L). Urinary sodium is increased. Which of the following is correct?

a. The patient's symptoms will be explained on the basis of folate deficiency
b. Only 50% of such patients will have parietal cell antibody
c. The patient is likely to have low levels of vitamin B_{12} and high levels of intrinsic factor
d. The patient is likely to have low levels of vitamin B_{12} and decreased secretion of intrinsic factor

342. In addition to anemia, this patient is most likely to have

a. Addison's disease of autoimmune etiology
b. Pituitary insufficiency
c. Hemochromatosis
d. Inappropriate ADH secretion

343. A 70-year-old intensive care unit patient complains of fever and shaking chills. The patient develops hypotension, and blood cultures are positive for gram-negative bacilli. The patient begins bleeding from venipuncture sites and around his Foley catheter. Laboratory studies are as follows:

Hct: 38%
WBC: 15,000/μL
Platelet count: 40,000/μL (normal 130,000 to 400,000)
Peripheral blood smear: fragmented RBCs
PT: elevated
PTT: elevated
Plasma fibrinogen: 70 mg/dL (normal 200 to 400)

The best course of therapy in this patient is

a. Begin heparin
b. Treat underlying disease
c. Begin plasmapheresis
d. Give vitamin K
e. Begin red blood cell transfusion

344. A 30-year-old female with Graves' disease has been started on propylthiouracil. She complains of low-grade fever, chills, and sore throat. The most important initial step in evaluating this patient's fever is

a. Serum TSH
b. Serum T_3
c. CBC
d. Chest x-ray
e. Blood cultures

Items 345–347

Match the clinical description with the most likely diagnosis.

a. Sideroblastic anemia
b. Thalassemia
c. Iron-deficiency anemia
d. Anemia of renal disease
e. Anemia of chronic disease

345. An alcoholic patient being treated for tuberculosis has an increase in serum iron and transferrin saturation. **(CHOOSE 1 DIAGNOSIS)**

346. A 70-year-old Hispanic woman presents with weight loss, constipation, and heme-positive stools. She has a microcytic anemia with low serum iron and elevated iron-binding capacity. **(CHOOSE 1 DIAGNOSIS)**

347. A 52-year-old African American diabetic requires hemodialysis for end-stage renal disease. She has hemoglobin of 9, hematocrit of 27, and normal red cell indices. The iron and iron-binding capacity are normal. **(CHOOSE 1 DIAGNOSIS)**

Items 348–351

Match the clinical description with the paraneoplastic syndrome most often associated with it

a. Humoral hypercalcemia of malignancy
b. Hyponatremia due to inappropriate ADH secretion
c. Hypoglycemia due to IGF-2
d. Migratory thrombophlebitis due to procoagulant cytokines
e. Skin infiltration with T lymphocytes

348. A 61-year-old woman with a large retroperitoneal sarcoma **(CHOOSE 1 SYNDROME)**

349. A 76-year-old woman with weight loss, depression, and a 4-cm pancreatic mass **(CHOOSE 1 SYNDROME)**

350. A 48-year-old cigarette smoker with a 4-cm hilar mass; transbronchial biopsy reveals a squamous cell carcinoma **(CHOOSE 1 SYNDROME)**

351. A 58-year-old cigarette smoker who develops a cough, hemoptysis, and a 2-cm perihilar density; sputum cytology shows small, undifferentiated cells **(CHOOSE 1 SYNDROME)**

352. A 64-year-old African American man presents for evaluation of a painless "lump" in the left thigh. He first noticed the abnormality about 1 month previously and thinks it has increased in size; there is no prior history of trauma. On exam, you find a 5-cm soft tissue mass, firm to hard in consistency, in the soft tissue above the knee. There is no tenderness or erythema; the mass is deep to the subcutaneous tissue and appears fixed to the underlying musculature. Inguinal lymph nodes are normal. You should

a. Reexamine the lesion in 3 months, as it is probably a lipoma
b. Obtain a bone scan
c. Treat with cephalexin 500 mg po qid for presumed abscess
d. Refer the patient for surgical biopsy

Hematology and Oncology

Answers

308. The answer is c. (*Braunwald, 15/e, pp 662–664.*) The patient has a microcytic anemia. A low serum iron, low ferritin, and high iron-binding capacity all suggest iron-deficiency anemia. Most iron-deficiency anemia is explained by blood loss. The patient's symptoms of constipation point to blood loss from the lower GI tract. Colonoscopy would be the highest-yield procedure. Barium enema misses 50% of polyps and a significant minority of colon cancers. Even patients without a history of GI symptoms who have no obvious explanation for their iron deficiency (such as menstrual blood loss or multiple prior pregnancies in women) should be studied for GI blood loss. Lead poisoning can cause a microcytic hypochromic anemia, but this would not be associated with the abnormal iron studies and low ferritin seen in this patient. Basophilic stippling or target cells seen on the peripheral blood smear would be important clues to the presence of lead poisoning. Folate deficiency presents as a megaloblastic anemia with macrocytosis (large, oval-shaped red cells) and hypersegmentation of the polymorphonuclear leukocytes.

309. The answer is c. (*Braunwald, 15/e, p 665.*) Patients with chronic inflammatory or neoplastic disease often develop anemia of chronic disease. Cytokines produced by inflammation cause a block in the normal recirculation of iron from reticuloendothelial cells (which pick up the iron from senescent red blood cells) to the red cell precursors (normoblasts). In addition, IL-1 and interferon γ decrease the production of and the response to erythropoietin. This causes a drop in the serum iron concentration and a normocytic or mild microcytic anemia. The inflammatory reaction, however, also decreases the iron-binding capacity (as opposed to iron-deficiency anemia, where the iron-binding capacity is elevated), so the saturation is usually between 10 and 20%. The anemia is rarely severe (Hb rarely less than 8.5 g/dL). The hemoglobin and hematocrit will improve if the underlying process is treated. Diseases not associated with inflammation or neoplasia (i.e., congestive heart failure, diabetes, hypertension, etc.) do not cause anemia of chronic disease. Blood loss would generally cause a lower serum iron level, an elevated iron-binding capacity, and a lower iron saturation. The serum ferritin (low in iron deficiency, normal or high in anemia of chronic disease) will usually clarify this situation. Vitamin B_{12} or folate deficiency are associated with a macrocytic anemia. Sideroblastic anemia can be either microcytic or macrocytic (occasionally with a dimorphic population of cells: some small and some large), but is not associated with a low iron level. In addition, this patient's history (which suggests an inflammatory polyarthritis) would not be consistent with sideroblastic anemia. The diagnosis of sideroblastic anemia is made by seeing ringed sideroblasts on bone marrow aspirate.

310. The answer is b. *(Braunwald, 15/e, pp 681, 686–689.)* An elevated reticulocyte count suggests active bone marrow response either to red blood cell loss (acute bleeding) or destruction (hemolysis). Many cases of hemolytic anemia can be diagnosed from changes on the peripheral blood smear. Large polychromatophilic cells suggest reticulocytes (which can be diagnosed with a reticulum stain). Microspherocytes suggest immune-mediated hemolysis. Fragmented cells suggest microvascular damage. This patient likely has immune-mediated hemolysis due to her *Mycoplasma* infection. This is usually associated with IgM antibodies, which react better at temperatures less than 37°C (and thus are called cold-reacting antibodies). The cold agglutinins associated with *Mycoplasma* typically react with anti-I cells. Those seen in infectious mononucleosis typically react with anti-i cells. Although the serum bilirubin and LDH are often elevated in hemolysis, they are less specific and tests would usually be performed after the reticulocyte count and peripheral blood smear. The *Mycoplasma* antigen test would confirm recent infection with *M. pneumoniae* but would not specifically explain the cause of the anemia.

311. The answer is a. *(Braunwald, 15/e, pp 727–733.)* The onset of multiple myeloma is usually insidious, with weakness and fatigue. Pain caused by bone involvement, anemia, renal insufficiency, and bacterial pneumonia often follow. This patient presented with fatigue and bone pain, then developed bacterial pneumonia probably secondary to *Streptococcus pneumoniae*, an encapsulated organism for which antibody to the polysaccharide capsule is not adequately produced by the myeloma patient. There is also evidence for renal insufficiency. Hypercalcemia is frequently seen in patients with multiple myeloma and may be life-threatening. Lymphoma typically presents with lymphadenopathy. Bone pain and renal insufficiency at the outset are uncommon; only the rare T cell lymphomas are commonly associated with hypercalcemia. Metastatic bronchogenic carcinoma can cause hypercalcemia but would rarely present with renal insufficiency and such severe anemia. Primary hyperparathyroidism is a common cause of hypercalcemia, but patients are usually minimally symptomatic. It does not cause severe anemia or increased incidence of infection.

312. The answer is b. (*Braunwald, 15/e, pp 727–733.*) Definitive diagnosis of multiple myeloma is made by demonstrating greater than 10% plasma cells in the bone marrow. None of the other findings are specific enough for definitive diagnosis. Renal biopsy would not be helpful. About 75% of patients with myeloma will have a monoclonal M spike on serum protein electrophoresis, but about 25% will produce primarily Bence-Jones proteins, which, because of their small size, do not accumulate in the serum but are excreted in the urine. A urine protein electrophoresis will identify these patients. Less than 1% of patients with myeloma will present with a nonsecretory myeloma; the diagnosis can only be made with bone marrow biopsy. Renal biopsy might show monoclonal protein deposition in the kidney or intratubular casts but would not be the first diagnostic procedure. Rouleaux formation, although characteristic of myeloma, is neither sensitive nor specific.

313. The answer is e. (*Braunwald, 15/e, pp 729, 732, 1544.*) Renal failure occurs in about 25% of myeloma patients, but many more have evidence of renal pathology. All factors listed may play a role in renal insufficiency; in addition, acute and chronic pyelonephritis frequently occur. Almost all patients with myeloma kidney, however, have evidence of tubular damage associated with the overexcretion of light chains. Light chains can be excreted at the rate of many grams per day, but nephrotic syndrome with edema and hypoalbuminemia do not occur because the proteins are globulins and not albumin (except in the unusual case of renal amyloidosis associated with myeloma). The light chain excretion causes primarily tubular rather than glomerular damage.

314. The answer is d. (*Braunwald, 15/e, pp 674–680.*) These neurologic deficits occur with vitamin B_{12} deficiency. This patient has a deficit of intrinsic factor after gastric surgery. Intrinsic factor is produced by gastric parietal cells and is a major factor in enhancing ileal absorption of B_{12}.

Milder degrees of B_{12} malabsorption can occur after partial gastrectomy, probably due to decreased release of B_{12} from food. Folic acid deficiency causes identical megaloblastic changes in the blood but is not associated with the neurologic deficit (loss of proprioception) that occurs with B_{12} deficiency. Thiamine deficiency causes beriberi; Vitamin K deficiency causes a coagulopathy associated with ecchymoses and prolongation of prothrombin time. These vitamins do not depend on gastric factors for their absorption.

315. The answer is c. *(Braunwald, 15/e, pp 715–721.)* Chronic lymphocytic leukemia is the most common of all leukemias, with incidence increasing with age. Patients are usually asymptomatic, but may complain of weakness, fatigue, or enlarged lymph nodes. The diagnosis is made by peripheral blood smear, as mature small lymphocytes constitute almost all the white blood cells seen. No other process produces a lymphocytosis of this morphology and magnitude. The leukemic cells in acute leukemia are immature blast cells that are easily distinguished from the normal-appearing mature lymphocytes of CLL. Both chronic myelogenous leukemia and the leukemoid reaction associated with illness such as TB are associated with increased numbers of a variety of cells of the myeloid series (mature polymorphonuclear leukocytes, metamyelocytes, myelocytes, etc.). The peripheral blood is said to resemble a dilute preparation of bone marrow. The presence of basophilia would suggest CML.

316. The answer is c. *(Braunwald, 15/e, pp 715–726.)* The commonly used Rai staging system for CLL begins with stage 0 (low-risk) CLL, which is associated with peripheral lymphocytosis alone. The patient with peripheral lymphadenopathy alone is at stage I. The presence of splenomegaly puts the patient in stage II (stages I and II are considered intermediate-risk). Stage III patients have an associated anemia, while stage IV is associated with thrombocytopenia (patients at stage III and IV are at high risk of complication and have a median survival of 1.5 years). Early treatment of CLL does not improve survival, and so treatment is usually reserved for symptomatic disease (bulky lyphadenopathy or splenomegaly) or high-risk disease (anemia and thrombocytopenia). Antimetabolites such as fludarabine and the alkylating agent chlorambucil are cornerstones of treatment. Steroids and immunoglobulin replacement may be used in patients with autoimmune cytopenias or symptomatic hypoglobulinemia (respectively).

317. The answer is b. *(Braunwald, 15/e, pp 562–571.)* Cigarette smokers have a 15- to 25-fold increased incidence of both squamous cell carcinoma and small cell undifferentiated carcinoma of the lung. Both of these neoplasms tend to be central (i.e., perihilar); the presence of obstructive lung disease increases the risk of lung cancer over and above the smoking history. Of the choices given, squamous cell carcinoma is the likeliest explanation for this patient's hemoptysis. Bronchoscopy would likely show the lesion and allow a tissue diagnosis to be made. Adenocarcinoma of the lung is the commonest lung cancer seen in nonsmokers, women, and younger patients. Its incidence is increased in smokers (probably twofold), but not to the degree seen with squamous cell carcinoma and small cell undifferentiated carcinoma. Adenocarcinoma is typically peripheral with pleural involvement (rather than the central involvement seen in this case). Bronchoalveolar cell carcinoma arises from alveolar epithelium, is typically peripheral, and may resemble a nonhealing pneumonia (it may even have air bronchograms like a pneumonia). Bronchial adenomas (carcinoid being the commonest type) are often central but are usually smaller and are less common than squamous cell carcinomas. Their incidence is not increased by cigarette smoking.

318. The answer is c. *(Braunwald, 15/e, pp 692–698.)* This patient has an unexplained pancytopenia. If all three elements (red blood cells, white blood cells, and platelets) are affected, the cause is usually in the bone marrow (although peripheral destruction from hypersplenism can occasionally cause pancytopenia). In this patient without a history of liver disease or palpable splenomegaly on physical examination, a bone marrow production problem is the most likely culprit. Although B_{12} deficiency can cause pancytopenia, usually a macrocytic anemia is the most prominent feature; a serum B_{12} level would be reasonable, but the most productive approach would be to examine the bone marrow. Leukemia can present without leukocytosis (so-called aleukemic leukemia), but the most likely diagnosis would be aplastic anemia. In the elderly patient, myelodysplastic syndrome (MDS) may present with pancytopenia.

319. The answer is b. *(Braunwald, 15/e, pp 620–622.)* The first step in this patient's evaluation is a pelvic exam to check for ovarian cancer. Pelvic fullness, vague discomfort, constipation, and early satiety are often the first symptoms of this disease. Ascites may be present on initial evaluation.

Abdominal ultrasound would follow. The CA 125 cancer antigen supports the diagnosis of ovarian cancer, but it is not sensitive or specific. If the pelvic exam and ultrasound were negative, sigmoidoscopy might be indicated to evaluate the patient's constipation.

320. The answer is a. (*Braunwald, 15/e, pp 620–622.*) Most ovarian cancers arise from the epithelium that covers the ovary (not the stroma or germ cells inside the ovary). Ovarian cancer is the leading cause of death from gynecological malignancy. Risk factors include infertility and frequent miscarriages. Pregnancy decreases the risk of ovarian cancer; each pregnancy decreases the risk by about 10%. Oral contraceptives appear to be protective as well. A family history of ovarian cancer is a major risk factor, increasing a woman's risk threefold. Patients with multiple affected first-degree relatives may carry the *BRCA1* or *BRCA2* genes. Coitus early in life and multiple partners are risk factors for cervical, but not ovarian, carcinoma.

321. The answer is b. (*Braunwald, 15/e, pp 605–608.*) Renal carcinoma is twice as common in men as women and tends to occur in the 50- to 70-year age group. Many patients present with a hematuria or flank pain, but the classic triad of hematuria, flank pain, and a palpable flank mass occurs in only 10 to 20% of patients. Paraneoplastic syndromes such as erythrocytosis, hypercalcemia, hepatic dysfunction, and fever of unknown origin are common. Surgery is the only potentially curable therapy; the results of treatment with chemotherapy or radiation therapy for nonresectable disease have been disappointing. Interferon α and interleukin 2 produce responses (but no cures) in 10 to 20% of patients. The prognosis for metastatic renal cell carcinoma is dismal.

322. The answer is a. (*Braunwald, 15/e, pp 606–608.*) Radical nephrectomy, including removal of the kidney, the surrounding fascia, the adrenal gland, and regional lymph nodes, provides the best chance for cure in patients with renal cell carcinoma. Partial (nephron-sparing) nephrectomy is being studied in selected cases. Radiation therapy is used in metastatic renal carcinoma, but results are disappointing. Immunotherapies such as interferon and interleukin 2 have been used for palliation.

323. The answer is a. (*Braunwald, 15/e, pp 617, 2146.*) The first step in evaluating a scrotal mass is to determine whether the mass is in the testis or outside it. Most solid masses arising from within the testis are malignant. Palpation of the scrotal mass and transillumination (holding a flashlight directly against the posterior wall of the scrotum) will distinguish testicular lesions from other masses within the scrotum, such as hydrocele. Ultrasonography will confirm a solid testicular mass. The tumor markers β-HCG and α-fetoprotein are not used in the initial evaluation of a scrotal mass, but may be important when a solid mass suggestive of testicular carcinoma is found. β-HCG or AFP will be elevated in about 70% of patients with disseminated nonseminomatous testicular cancer. Seminomas are usually associated with normal tumor cell markers. Choriocarcinomas produce β-HCG. Endodermal sinus tumors or embryonal cell carcinomas are often associated with elevated AFP levels. The lymphatic drainage of the testis is into the periaortic nodes, not to the inguinal nodes. The periaortic nodes must be assessed radiographically, usually by CT scanning, if a testicular neoplasm is strongly suspected.

324. The answer is d. (*Braunwald, 15/e, pp 604–606.*) Unexplained gross hematuria requires evaluation. Patients who have gross hematuria in association with clear-cut urinary tract infection are usually treated and followed with a repeat urinalysis to confirm clearing of the RBCs, but this patient has no symptoms of urinary tract infection. Although benign causes (prostatitis, renal stones) are most common, as many as 30% of patients with gross hematuria will have malignancies of the genitourinary tract. Cigarette smoking increases the risk of bladder cancer two- to four-fold. Exposure to aniline dyes, chronic cyclophosphamide treatment, external beam radiation, and *Schistosoma* infection of the bladder are other risk factors. This patient should be referred to a urologist for cystoscopy to rule out transitional cell carcinoma of the bladder. If no lesion is found, CT scanning of the kidneys would be indicated despite the previous negative sonogram.

325. The answer is a. (*Braunwald, 15/e, pp 360–1365.*) The long-term nature of these symptoms, the fact that the nodes are nontender, and their location (including scalene and supraclavicular) all suggest the likelihood of malignancy. Although infectious mononucleosis and toxoplasmosis can cause diffuse lymphadenopathy, these infections are usually associated with other evidence of infection such as pharyngitis, fever, and atypical lymphocytosis in the peripheral blood. It would be unusual for the lymphadenopathy associated with these infections to persist for 2 months. Serum angiotensin converting enzyme level is a nonspecific test for sarcoidosis but is also elevated in other granulomatous diseases and is not sensitive or specific enough to be used as an initial diagnostic test. Lymphadenopathy associated with sarcoidosis requires a biopsy for diagnosis. In this patient, an excisional biopsy is necessary primarily to rule out the malignancy, particularly lymphoma.

326. The answer is a. (*Braunwald, 15/e, pp 725–726.*) The staging of Hodgkin's disease is important so that proper treatment can be planned. Stage I (single lymph node bearing area) or stage II (more than one lymph node site on the same side of the diaphragm) patients who have good prognostic features may be treated with radiation therapy. Those with stage III (affected lymph nodes on both sides of the diaphragm) or stage IV (extranodal disease) are treated with combination chemotherapy. A CT scan or an MRI of the abdomen will show evidence of lymph node involvement below the diaphragm. Staging laparotomy with splenectomy, formerly done to provide pathology of the periaortic nodes and spleen, is rarely done today. Gallium scans can be useful in difficult cases. Bone marrow biopsy is usually performed to exclude bone marrow disease, which would imply stage IV.

327. The answer is b. (*Braunwald, 15/e, pp 608–616.*) A prostate biopsy is necessary to confirm the diagnosis of prostatic carcinoma. A metastatic workup, including bone scan, would then follow. Bone scan is a very sensitive test for metastatic prostate carcinoma, which tends to spread through the venous plexus surrounding the prostate to the sacrum and lower lumbar vertebrae. Since prostate cancer stimulates osteoblastic activity of the bone, and since osteoblasts (rather than osteoclasts) take up the tracer used in bone scanning, the test is very reliable. Pure osteolytic metastases (typically seen in myeloma, occasionally in thyroid or renal carcinoma) will not produce hot spots on bone scans. CT scanning of pelvic nodes is occasionally used to assess resectability. If this patient has bony metastases, however, systemic rather than local therapy will be necessary.

328. The answer is d. (*Braunwald 15/e, pp 608–613.*) Patients with metastatic prostatic carcinoma are treated with endocrine therapy to shrink primary and secondary lesions by depriving prostatic tissue of circulating androgens. Estrogens are no longer recommended because of the high incidence of cardiovascular events. Most patients now receive a GnRH analogue or surgical castration; whether an antiandrogen (such as flutamide) provides additional benefit is currently a matter of debate. Radiotherapy is used for localized disease, but is less effective than hormonal therapy. No effective chemotherapy is currently available.

329. The answer is c. *(Braunwald, 15/e, pp 745–746.)* Heparin is the commonest cause of drug-induced thrombocytopenia. Between 10 and 15% of patients receiving unfractionated heparin develop thrombocytopenia. The drop in platelet count is due to the production of an antibody against a complex of heparin and platelet factor 4. Low-molecular-weight heparin can also cause thrombocytopenia, although less frequently than unfractionated heparin. Although a bone marrow study to show the presence of megakaryocytes is occasionally indicated in unexplained thrombocytopenia, in this patient with a history strongly suggestive of a drug-induced thrombocytopenia, a bone marrow examination would not be necessary. The diagnosis of idiopathic thrombocytopenic purpura requires the exclusion of drugs likely to cause a decline in the platelet count. Other drugs that may cause thrombocytopenia include chemotherapeutic agents, antibiotics such as sulfonamides and β-lactams, and cardiovascular agents including thiazide diuretics or quinidine.

330. The answer is c. *(Braunwald, 15/e, pp 746, 758.)* Heparin-induced thrombocytopenia causes a white clot syndrome rather than bleeding (which is uncommon in HIT). The patient develops platelet aggregation and excess clotting, which can be either venous or arterial. Patients may develop stroke, myocardial infarction, digital gangrene, etc. Although HIT usually resolves spontaneously after 7 to 10 days, the development of thrombosis due to HIT requires therapy with alternative anticoagulants. Although low-molecular-weight heparin infrequently causes HIT, its use is contraindicated in the white clot syndrome. The administration of either lepirudin (a direct thrombin antagonist) or danaparoid (a heparinoid that does not cause HIT) can be lifesaving. Warfarin is used long-term, but only after lepirudin or danaproid has been instituted. Although the lupus anticoagulant can cause both venous and arterial thrombosis, this patient likely has a drug-induced thrombocytopenia. The lupus anticoagulant often occurs in the absence of clinical lupus; therefore, an ANA would not be indicated.

331. The answer is c. (*Braunwald, 15/e, pp 426–428.*) Rifampin induces the cytochrome P450 that metabolizes warfarin; higher doses of warfarin are required to overcome this effect. When rifampin is stopped, the dose of warfarin necessary to produce a therapeutic prothrombin time will decrease. Barbiturates also accelerate the metabolism of warfarin. Many drugs interfere with the metabolism and clearance of warfarin. Drugs such as nonsteroidal anti-inflammatories can compete with warfarin for albumin-binding sites and will lead to an increased prothrombin time. The list of medications that can either increase or decrease the effect of warfarin is long; all patients given this drug should be advised to contact their physician before taking any new drug. They should also be counseled about over-the-counter drugs (aspirin and NSAIDs) or even health food supplements (such as Ginkgo biloba) that can also affect the prothrombin time in these patients.

332. The answer is b. (*Braunwald, 15/e, pp 2259–2260.*) Patients with hemochromatosis and cirrhosis have a very high incidence of hepatocellular carcinoma. The incidence of this complication is 30% and increases with age. Weight loss and abdominal pain suggest hepatoma in this patient. A CT scan or ultrasound would be indicated. The picture of right upper quadrant pain and elevated alkaline phosphatase would not suggest acute hepatitis (which causes an elevation of the transaminases) or worsening of the cirrhosis caused by hemochromatosis. Primary biliary cirrhosis can cause an obstructive biliary disease, but would be much less likely in this patient.

333. The answer is c. (*Braunwald, 15/e, p 560.*) The lesion described is characteristic of leukoplakia. This is a precancerous lesion that requires biopsy. Histologically, these lesions show hyperkeratosis, acanthosis, and atypia. There are homogeneous and nonhomogeneous types; the homogeneous are much more likely to undergo malignant transformation. Oropharyngeal *Candida* would be unlikely to occur in this patient and would appear as a more diffuse, lacy lesion of the buccal mucosa and oropharynx. The white plaque of thrush would rub off, leaving a slightly erythematous and inflamed mucosa underneath.

334–338. The answers are 334-a, 335-d, 336-c, 337-a, 338-b. (*Braunwald, 15/e, pp 554–557, 617, 622, 706, 743.*) Most cancers are cured only when found in an early or localized state. A few malignancies, however, are curable even when distant metastases are present. Among these are gestational choriocarcinoma, certain acute leukemias, and certain lymphomas. The demonstration that testicular carcinoma is curable by combination chemotherapy represented a major advance in the treatment of this neoplasm. Seminomas are quite sensitive to radiation therapy, but even non-seminomatous tumors are curable with platinum-based chemotherapy. Metastases beyond the retroperitoneal nodes, very high α-fetoprotein or β-HCG levels, or LDH levels above 10 times normal confer poor prognosis, but even these patients can be cured 50% of the time.

Metastatic melanoma is a devastating disease with 5-year survival of less than 10%. The only curative strategy for melanoma is surgery when the disease is localized (preferably to the skin, although 50% of those with one metastatic regional node can be cured with local excision and lymph node dissection). Chemotherapy produces partial response in less than 20% of these patients. Interferon and interleukin 2 are used with similarly disappointing results.

Breast cancer that has metastasized beyond the axillary lymph nodes is an incurable disease; however, many forms of therapy lead to complete remission in 30 to 40% of patients treated. Patients who are estrogen receptor–positive are often treated with hormone-based regimens. ER-negative and younger women usually receive doxorubicin-based treatment. In addition, bone metastases can be palliated with diphosphonates. Even extensive Hodgkin's disease is a curable malignancy. Although radiation therapy is occasionally used for localized disease, most patients are treated with combination chemotherapy with good response. Nitrogen mustard, vincristine, prednisone, and procarbazine (MOPP) was the first combination chemotherapy that was proven to cure even advanced Hodgkin's disease. Most patients now are treated with adriamycin, bleomycin, vinblastine, and dacarbazine (ABVD). Even in stage IV disease, 50 to 70% of patients should be cured.

Small cell undifferentiated (oat cell) carcinoma of the lung is sensitive both to radiation and chemotherapy, but once the disease has spread beyond the involved hemithorax it is rarely curable. Before effective treatment was available, most patients with this aggressive neoplasm survived between 2 and 3 months. With combination chemotherapy, anticipated survival is 1 to 2 years. A combination of etoposide and a platinum derivative is usually used. Due to the impermeability of the blood-brain barrier to many chemotherapeutic agents, radiation therapy is necessary for brain metastases. Although an occasional patient with extensive oat cell carcinoma is cured, prolongation of survival is the anticipated outcome.

339. The answer is c. (*Braunwald, 15/e, pp 669–671.*) Splenomegaly is not typical of sickle cell anemia. Recurrent splenic infarcts usually occur during childhood and lead to a small, infarcted spleen with functional asplenia. These patients often have Howell-Jolly bodies on peripheral blood smear (indicative of asplenia) and have an increased incidence of infection with encapsulated organisms. The presence of an enlarged spleen in a patient with sickle cells on peripheral blood smear is most often seen in hemoglobin SC disease. The state of hemolysis results in an unconjugated hyperbilirubinemia and low-grade icterus. Anemia and hypoxemia result in a hyperdynamic circulation and a systolic ejection murmur. Ankle ulcers and other chronic skin ulcers may be persistent problems, particularly in those with severe anemia.

340. The answer is e. (*Braunwald, 15/e, pp 685–686.*) This patient has developed a hemolytic anemia secondary to an antimalarial drug. Toxins or drugs such as primaquine, sulfamethoxazole, and nitrofurantoin cause hemolysis in patients with G6PD deficiency. It occurs most commonly in African Americans; since the G6PD gene is carried on the X chromosome, most affected patients are males. The drugs that cause hemolysis in G6PD deficiency are oxidizing agents. Oxidant stress on red blood cells is counteracted by reduced glutathione. NADPH (which is required to regenerate reduced glutathione after it has been oxidized) is produced by the hexose monophosphate shunt. G6PD is the first enzyme in this metabolic pathway. If this enzyme is less active, the cell cannot replace GSH and succumbs to oxidizing stress. Clinically this can range from mild to life-threatening hemolysis. In mild cases, no treatment is necessary; once the offending drug is eliminated, the hemolysis resolves.

341. The answer is d. (*Braunwald, 15/e, pp 674–680.*) With anemia and hypersegmented polyps, this patient has a megaloblastic anemia. The evidence for neuropathy makes B_{12} deficiency the diagnosis, since folate deficiency does not cause neuropathy. Pernicious anemia with low B_{12} levels and decreased secretion of intrinsic factor is the most likely cause, although B_{12} deficiency from intestinal malabsorption cannot be ruled out. Antiparietal antibody occurs in 90% of patients with pernicious anemia.

342. The answer is a. (*Braunwald, 15/e, pp 2189–2190.*) The patient has signs and symptoms of adrenal insufficiency, including postural hypotension, hyperpigmentation, hyponatremia, and hyperkalemia. The incidence of pernicious anemia is increased in patients with other autoimmune diseases, such as idiopathic adrenal insufficiency (Addison's disease), Graves' disease, and hypothyroidism. Vitiligo is also common in these patients and is due to autoimmune destruction of melanocytes. Inappropriate ADH secretion can cause hypoatremia, but it does not cause volume depletion (i.e., postural hypotension) or hyperkalemia. Hemochromatosis can cause skin hyperpigmentation but is not associated with anemia or adrenal insufficiency.

343. The answer is b. (*Braunwald, 15/e, pp 754–755.*) This patient with gram-negative bacteremia has developed disseminated intravascular coagulation, as evidenced by multiple-site bleeding, thrombocytopenia, fragmented red blood cells on peripheral smear, prolonged PT and PTT, and reduced fibrinogen levels from depletion of coagulation proteins. Initial treatment is directed at correcting the underlying disorder—in this case infection. Although heparin was formerly recommended for the treatment of DIC, it is now used rarely and only in unusual circumstances (such as acute promyelocytic leukemia). For the patient who continues to bleed, supplementation of platelets and clotting factors (with fresh frozen plasma or cryoprecipitate) may help control life-threatening bleeding. Red cell fragmentation and low platelet count can be seen in microangiopathic disorders such as TTP, but in these disorders the coagulation pathway is not activated. Therefore in TTP the prothrombin time and partial thromboplastin time as well as the plasma fibrinogen levels will be normal.

344. The answer is c. (*Braunwald, 15/e, pp 368–369, 432.*) Propylthiouracil can cause a mild leukopenia that does not require discontinuation of the drug. Drug-induced agranulocytosis is a life-threatening complication occurring in 0.1 to 0.2% of patients on antithyroid medications and requires immediate discontinuation of the drug. Agranulocytosis is an immune-mediated disorder; the absolute neutrophil count is often extremely depressed (usually less than 100). Generally the neutrophil count will recover 5 to 7 days after the offending drug has been discontinued. During this time the patient is at grave risk of septicemia. Although blood cultures are indicated in this patient prior to the administration of antibiotics, the most important initial step is evaluating the white blood cell count.

345–347. The answers are 345-a, 346-c, 347-d. *(Braunwald, 15/e, pp 660–667.)* The alcoholic patient being treated for tuberculosis has sideroblastic anemia. Both ethanol and isoniazid inhibit one or more steps in heme synthesis. The disorder results in ringed sideroblasts, nucleated erythroid precursors, a hypochromic microcytic anemia, and a characteristic increase in serum iron and transferrin saturation.

Both iron-deficiency anemia and anemia of chronic disease are associated with a low serum iron level. In iron-deficiency anemia, the TIBC is high and the iron saturation is usually less than 10%. In anemia of chronic disease, the iron-binding capacity is low and the saturation is usually between 10 and 20%. In borderline cases, a serum ferritin level will usually make the distinction (it is low in iron-deficiency anemia and normal or high in anemia of chronic disease). Both anemias can be normocytic if mild and microcytic if moderate in severity. Anemia of chronic disease is rarely severe (i.e., hemoglobin rarely below 8.5); a severe anemia associated with a very low MCV is usually iron deficiency or thalassemia.

The anemia of renal disease is normocytic and normochromic. The red cells themselves are normal but are not stimulated to proliferate due to inadequate amounts of erythropoietin. The diseased kidney is unable to produce adequate amounts of erythropoietin. Numbers of white cells and platelets are usually normal.

348–351. The answers are 348-c, 349-d, 350-a, 351-b. *(Braunwald, 15/e, pp 632–640.)* Tumor-induced hypoglycemia is a relatively rare paraneoplastic syndrome. True insulin production is uncommon; most true insulinomas are benign islet cell tumors of the pancreas. Occasionally a large retroperitoneal sarcoma will produce insulin-like growth factor 2, which can cause hypoglycemia with a very high rate of glucose use. Glucose infusions of 10 to 20 g/h may be required to treat the hypoglycemia.

The classic Trousseau syndrome consists of migratory superficial thrombophlebitis. A single episode of tenderness and inflammation in a superficial vein is common and usually benign, but recurrent unprovoked episodes should prompt a search for an underlying neoplasm. Cancer of the pancreas is the classic and commonest cancer, but any mucin-producing carcinoma can produce this syndrome.

Humoral hypercalcemia of malignancy resembles hyperparathyroidism, but the substance produced by the cancer is parathormone-related peptide (PTHrP), which does not cross-react with PTH on modern assays. PTHrP is an oncofetal protein involved in squamous differentiation in the fetus. For this reason squamous cancers (lung, head and neck, cervix) are the usual causes. Adenocarcinomas are relatively uncommon causes of this syndrome.

Oat cell (small cell undifferentiated) carcinomas of the lung arise from neuroendocrine cells and thus commonly produce ectopic hormones. ADH (vasopressin) is the commonest and causes hyponatremia, but production of ACTH (usually causing hypokalemia and muscle weakness rather than the classic full-blown Cushing syndrome) occurs frequently. Therefore a lung mass in association with either hyponatremia or hypokalemia suggests oat cell carcinoma.

352. The answer is d. *(Braunwald, 15/e, pp 625–628.)* Although lipomas are the commonest soft tissue mass, they are soft and mobile with the subcutaneous tissue and grow very slowly. Any atypical or enlarging soft tissue mass should be further evaluated, either by CT or MRI scan or by biopsy, because this is how soft tissue sarcomas present. The size, firmness, and fixity to deep tissues are all worrisome features in this patient, and a biopsy should be requested even if the CT scan is reassuring; therefore, open biopsy would be the preferred approach. Sixty percent of soft tissue sarcomas arise in the extremities, with the lower extremities three times as common as the upper extremities. A variety of histological types are possible and are not predictable from clinical features, although malignant fibrous histiocytomas are most common. The only curative approach is complete surgical resection. Radiation and chemotherapy have a role in adjuvant or palliative therapy. Occasional patients with favorable metastatic disease enter long-term remission with aggressive therapy. Soft tissue sarcomas metastasize hematogenously, most often to the lungs; lymph node metastases would not be expected.

Neurology

Questions

DIRECTIONS: Each item below contains a question or incomplete statement followed by suggested responses. Select the **one best** response to each question.

353. A 30-year-old male complains of unilateral headaches with rhinorrhea and tearing of the eye on the side of the headache. Episodes are precipitated by alcohol. Headaches may become a problem for weeks to months, after which a headache-free period occurs. The most likely diagnosis is

a. Migraine
b. Cluster headache
c. Sinusitis
d. Tension headache

354. A 35-year-old previously healthy woman complains of a severe, excruciating headache and then has a transient loss of consciousness. There are no focal neurologic findings. The next step in evaluation is

a. CT scan without contrast
b. CT scan with contrast
c. Carotid angiogram
d. Holter monitor

355. A 70-year-old male complains of the sudden onset of syncope. It occurs without warning and with no sweating, dizziness, or light-headedness. He believes episodes tend to occur when he turns his head too quickly or sometimes when he is shaving. The best way to make a definitive diagnosis in this patient is

a. ECG
b. Carotid massage with ECG monitoring
c. Holter monitor
d. Electrophysiologic studies to evaluate the AV node

Items 356–358

356. A 30-year-old male complains of leg weakness and paresthesias of the arm and leg. Five years previously he had an episode of transient visual loss. On physical exam, there is hyperreflexia, bilateral Babinski signs, and cerebellar dysmetria with poor finger-to-nose movement. When the patient is asked to look to the right, the left eye does not move normally past the midline. Nystagmus is noted in the abducting eye. A more detailed history suggests the patient has had several episodes of gait difficulty that have resolved spontaneously. He appears to be stable between these episodes. He has no systemic symptoms of fever or weight loss. The most likely diagnosis in this patient is

a. Multiple sclerosis
b. Vitamin B_{12} deficiency
c. Systemic lupus erythematosus
d. Hypochondriasis

357. The best test to pursue this diagnosis is

a. Lumbar puncture
b. MRI
c. Quantitative IgG levels
d. Oligoclonal banding

358. Which of the following best summarizes the role of interferon β for this disease?

a. It can reduce the number of relapses and the appearance of new lesions on MRI
b. It can cure one-third of patients
c. It improves survival
d. It improves patients' symptoms and has no significant side effects

Items 359–360

359. A 50-year-old male complains of slowly progressive weakness over several months. Walking has become more difficult, as has using his hands. There are no sensory, bowel, or bladder complaints, or any problems in thinking, speech, or vision. Examination shows distal muscle weakness with muscle wasting and fasciculations. There are also upper motor neuron signs, including extensor plantar reflexes and hyperreflexia in wasted muscle groups. The most likely diagnosis is

a. Polymyositis
b. Duchenne muscular dystrophy
c. Amyotrophic lateral sclerosis
d. Myasthenia gravis

360. The laboratory test most likely to be abnormal in this patient is

a. Cerebrospinal fluid white blood cell count
b. Sensory conduction studies
c. CT scan of the brain
d. Electromyography

361. Which of the following is correct with respect to treatment of this patient?

a. Riluzole arrests the underlying pathologic process in ALS
b. Riluzole was FDA approved for ALS because it improves survival rate
c. Riluzole has no significant side effects
d. Insulin-like growth factor is another alternative for the treatment of ALS

362. A 20-year-old woman complains of weakness that is worse in the afternoon, worse during repetitive activity, and improved by rest. When fatigued, the patient is unable to hold her head up, speak, or chew her food. On physical exam, there is no loss of reflexes, sensation, or coordination. The underlying pathogenesis of this disease is

a. Serum antiacetylcholine receptor antibodies causing neuromuscular transmission failure
b. Destruction of anterior horn cells by virus
c. Progressive muscular atrophy
d. Demyelinating disease

363. The diagnosis of myasthenia gravis is made by a positive edrophonium test, repetitive nerve stimulation test of a weak muscle, and anti-acetylcholine receptor antibody assay. MRI of the mediastinum is now indicated to

a. Rule out tuberculosis before starting prednisone
b. Rule out thymoma
c. Look for small cell carcinoma and Lambert-Eaton syndrome
d. Rule out sarcoidosis

DIRECTIONS: Each group of questions below consists of lettered options followed by a set of numbered items. For each numbered item, select the **one** lettered option with which it is **most** closely associated. Each lettered option may be used once, more than once, or not at all.

Items 364–366

Match the clinical description with the most likely disease process.

a. Parkinson's disease
b. Wilson's disease
c. Huntington's chorea
d. Dystonia
e. Essential tremor
f. Tic

364. An 18-year-old male with resting tremor, bradykinesia, rigidity, drooling; deposits in cornea; and abnormal liver function tests **(CHOOSE 1 DISEASE PROCESS)**

365. An elderly patient with bradykinesia, micrographia, and resting tremor **(CHOOSE 1 DISEASE PROCESS)**

366. Rapid, writhing movements in a 40-year-old associated with dementia **(CHOOSE 1 DISEASE PROCESS)**

Items 367–368

367. Three weeks after an upper respiratory illness, a 25-year-old male develops weakness of his arms and legs over several days. On physical exam he is tachypneic, with shallow respirations and symmetric muscle weakness in both arms and legs. There is no obvious sensory deficit, but motor reflexes cannot be elicited. The most likely diagnosis is

a. Myasthenia gravis
b. Multiple sclerosis
c. Guillain-Barré syndrome
d. Dermatomyositis
e. Diabetes mellitus

368. The workup of this patient is most likely to show

a. Acellular spinal fluid with high protein
b. Abnormal EMG that shows axonal degeneration
c. Positive Tensilon test
d. Elevated CPK
e. Respiratory alkalosis by arterial blood gases

Items 369–372

For each of the clinical descriptions, select a diagnosis.

a. Senile dementia of the Alzheimer's type
b. Multi-infarct dementia
c. Vitamin B_{12} deficiency
d. Delirium
e. Creutzfeldt-Jakob disease
f. Normal pressure hydrocephalus

369. An 80-year-old develops steady, progressive memory and cognitive deficit over 2 years. He has normal blood pressure and no focal neurologic findings, and workup for dementia is negative. **(SELECT 1 DIAGNOSIS)**

370. A 60-year-old woman admitted for urinary retention develops acute confusion and disorientation. **(SELECT 1 DIAGNOSIS)**

371. A 70-year-old male with history of hypertension and previous history of stroke presents with new focal findings and acute worsening of cognitive function. (**SELECT 1 DIAGNOSIS**)

372. A 50-year-old presents with rapidly progressive change in mental status over 3 months, with episodes of myoclonus and abnormal EEG. (**SELECT 1 DIAGNOSIS**)

Items 373–375

Match each clinical description with the correct diagnosis.

a. Pneumococcal meningitis
b. Cryptococcal meningitis
c. Viral Meningitis
d. Brain abscess
e. Hemophilus influenzae meningitis

373. Fever, stiff neck; CSF has positive quellung reaction (**CHOOSE 1 DIAGNOSIS**)

374. Patient on high-dose corticosteroids; positive india ink stain (**CHOOSE 1 DIAGNOSIS**)

375. History of dental abscess; has focal neurologic findings and low-grade fever (**CHOOSE 1 DIAGNOSIS**)

Items 376–378

Match each symptom or sign with the appropriate diagnosis.

a. Tension headache
b. Cluster headache
c. Migraine headache
d. Temporal arteritis
e. Brain tumor
f. Sinusitis
g. Temporomandibular joint dysfunction
h. Tic doloureux

376. Bilateral, bandlike sensation around head; dull, steady pain that may last days, weeks; possible occipital or nuchal soreness **(SELECT 1 DIAGNOSIS)**

377. Unilateral, nonthrobbing headache; more common in men; nasal stuffiness and lacrimation **(SELECT 1 DIAGNOSIS)**

378. Unilateral headache with localized scalp tenderness in older patient; may have transient visual loss **(SELECT 1 DIAGNOSIS)**

379. A 45-year-old woman presents to her physician with an 8-month history of gradually increasing limb weakness. She first noticed difficulty climbing stairs, then problems rising from chairs, walking more than half a block, and, finally, lifting her arms above shoulder level. Aside from some difficulty swallowing, she has no ocular, bulbar, or sphincter problems and no sensory complaints. Family history is negative for neurological disease. Examination reveals significant proximal limb and neck muscle weakness with minimal atrophy, normal sensory findings, and intact deep tendon reflexes. The most likely diagnosis in this patient is

a. Polymyositis
b. Cervical myelopathy
c. Myasthenia gravis
d. Mononeuropathy multiplex
e. Limb-girdle muscular dystrophy

380. A 55-year-old diabetic woman suddenly develops weakness of the left side of her face as well as of her right arm and leg. She also has diplopia on left lateral gaze. The responsible lesion is probably located in the

a. Right cerebral hemisphere
b. Left cerebral hemisphere
c. Right side of the brainstem
d. Left side of the brainstem
e. Right medial longitudinal fasciculus

381. A 40-year-old woman complains of headache associated with visual disturbance. Of the histories described below, which one suggests migraine headache as a likely diagnosis?

a. Numbness or tingling of the left face, lips, and hand lasting for 5 to 15 min, followed by throbbing headache
b. An increasingly throbbing headache associated with unilateral visual loss and generalized muscle aches
c. A continuous headache associated with sleepiness, nausea, ataxia, and incoordination of the right upper limb
d. An intense left retroorbital headache associated with transient left-sided ptosis and rhinorrhea
e. A visual field defect that persists following cessation of a unilateral headache

382. A 60-year-old man with Parkinson's disease is receiving levodopa/cardiodopa therapy and complains of uncontrollable facial movements. Which of the following is correct?

a. Limb and facial dyskinesias are unusual side effects of chronic levodopa therapy
b. Levodopa treatment, while ameliorating symptoms, does not alter the natural history of the disease
c. Bromocriptine works by increasing the release of dopamine from the substantia nigra
d. Trihexyphenidyl and benztropine mesylate have minimal side effects in the elderly

Items 383–386

For each symptom, select the most likely type of seizure.

a. Absence (petit mal) seizure
b. Complex partial seizure
c. Simple partial seizure
d. Atonic seizure
e. Myoclonic seizure

383. Postictal confusion **(SELECT 1 SEIZURE TYPE)**

384. Three-per-second spike-and-wave discharges **(SELECT 1 SEIZURE TYPE)**

385. Déjà vu experiences **(SELECT 1 SEIZURE TYPE)**

386. Loss of postural muscle tone and brief loss of consciousness **(SELECT 1 SEIZURE TYPE)**

Item 387–390

For each symptom of cerebrovascular disease, select the site of the lesion.
a. Internal carotid artery
b. Middle cerebral artery
c. Midbasilar artery
d. Anterior cerebral artery
e. Penetrating branch, middle cerebral artery

387. Sudden, painless monocular blindness **(SELECT 1 LESION SITE)**

388. Unilateral or bilateral weakness, sensory loss, disorder of ocular motility, loss of facial sensation, ataxia **(SELECT 1 LESION SITE)**

389. Contralateral weakness and sensory loss, worse in face and arm; homonymous hemianopsia; aphasia or neglect syndrome **(SELECT 1 LESION SITE)**

390. Pure motor hemiparesis involving face, arm, and leg **(SELECT 1 LESION SITE)**

Neurology

Answers

353. The answer is b. (*Braunwald, 15/e, pp 70–71.*) This headache is most consistent with a type of neurovascular headache called cluster headache. These occur most often in young men; have a characteristic periodicity, or cluster; and cause lacrimation, nasal stuffiness, and sometimes conjunctival inflammation. Migraines tend not to come and go in this manner, are more throbbing, and are more likely to be associated with nausea and vomiting. Sinusitis is usually bilateral with associated fever and purulent discharge. Tension headaches are usually described as bandlike, without lacrimation or nasal congestion.

354. The answer is a. (*Stobo, 23/e, pp 849–850.*) An excruciating headache with syncope requires evaluation for subarachnoid hemorrhage. In about 80% of patients, there will be enough blood to be visualized on a noncontrast CT scan. If the scan is normal, a lumbar puncture is the next step to establish the presence of subarachnoid blood. A contrast CT scan sometimes obscures the diagnosis because, in an enhanced scan, normal arteries may be mistaken for clotted blood.

355. The answer is b. (*Braunwald, 15/e, p 112.*) When syncope occurs in an older patient as a result of head turning, wearing a tight shirt collar, or shaving over the neck area, carotid sinus hypersensitivity should be considered. It usually occurs in men above the age of 50. Baroreceptors of the carotid sinus are activated and pass impulses through the glossopharyngeal nerve to the medulla oblongata. Some consider the process to be quite rare. Gentle massage of one carotid sinus at a time may show a period of asystole. This should be performed in a controlled setting with monitoring and atropine available.

356. The answer is a. (*Braunwald, 15/e, pp 2454–2457.*) This patient's episode of transient blindness was likely due to optic neuritis. This transient loss of vision in one eye occurs in about 25 to 40% of multiple sclerosis patients. (A similar presentation can occur in SLE, sarcoidosis, or syphilis.)

In addition, the patient gives a history of a relapsing-remitting process. There are abnormal signs of cerebellar and upper motor neuron disease. Signs and symptoms therefore suggest multiple lesions, making multiple sclerosis the most likely diagnosis. There are no systemic symptoms to suggest SLE. B_{12} deficiency could not explain all of the neurologic findings, i.e., visual loss and cerebellar dysmetria. Objective physical exam data rules out hypochondriasis—a diagnosis sometimes inappropriately given to the MS patient.

357. The answer is b. *(Braunwald, 15/e, pp 2456–2457.)* All patients with suspected multiple sclerosis should have an MRI of the brain. MRI is sensitive in defining demyelinating lesions in the brain and spinal cord. Disease-related changes are found in over 95% of patients who have definite evidence for MS. Most patients do not need lumbar puncture or spinal fluid analysis for diagnosis, although 70% have elevated IgG levels and myelin basic protein does appear in the CSF during exacerbations. When the diagnosis is in doubt, lumbar puncture is indicated. Pleocytosis of greater than 75 cells per microliter or finding polymorphonuclear leukocytes in the CSF make the diagnosis of MS unlikely. In some cases, chronic infection such as with syphilis or HIV may be in the differential of MS. Quantitative IgG levels would not be specific enough for diagnosis. Oligoclonal banding of CSF IgG is determined by agarose gel electrophoresis. Two or more bands are found in 70 to 90% of patients with MS.

358. The answer is a. *(Braunwald, 15/e, pp 2457–2458.)* Both interferon β 1b and interferon β 1a are approved for use in patients with multiple sclerosis who have relapsing-remitting or progressive MS. Glatiramer acetate (Copaxone) is now also approved for MS. While patients who receive any one of these treatments have 30% fewer exacerbations and fewer new MRI lesions, the treatments do not cure the disease. Interferon β can cause side effects, particularly a flulike syndrome that resolves within several months.

359. The answer is c. *(Braunwald, 15/e, pp 2412–2414.)* The disease described involves motor neurons exclusively. Amyotrophic lateral sclerosis affects both upper and lower motor neurons. In this patient, there is upper and lower motor neuron involvement without sensory deficit. Lower motor neuron signs include focal weakness, focal wasting, and fasciculations. Upper motor neuron signs include an extensor plantar response and an increased tendon reflex in a weakened muscle. Peripheral neuropathy and dementia do not occur in ALS. Primary muscle diseases produce weakness by affecting muscle fibers without interfering with the nerve itself or the neuromuscular junction. Duchenne muscular dystrophy occurs at a younger age and involves proximal muscle weakness and not motor neurons. Polymyositis is also primarily a muscle disease. Myasthenia gravis would not cause hyperreflexia or Babinski reflex; it is a disease of muscle weakness characterized by fatigability.

360. The answer is d. *(Braunwald, 15/e, p 2414.)* EMG would show widespread denervation and fibrillation potentials with preserved nerve conduction velocities. There is no inflammatory reaction in the CSF. ALS does not involve sensory neurons. A CT or MRI of the brain could be used to rule out masses in the region of the foramen magnum. In some patients, a CT of the cervical spine might be needed to rule out a structural lesion of the spine, which could mimic ALS.

361. The answer is b. *(Braunwald, 15/e, pp 2414–2415.)* Riluzole is approved by the FDA for the treatment of ALS. It has been shown to moderately prolong life in the ALS patient, although it does not arrest the disease process. Its mechanism of action may be inhibition of the release of the neurotransmitter glutamate with reduction of excitotoxicity. The drug has several side effects including nausea, weight loss, and liver function abnormalities. Insulin-like growth factor (IGF-1) was shown to slow the progression of ALS in one study, but results were not confirmed in a second study and IGF-1 is not available as a treatment option at present.

362. The answer is a. *(Braunwald, 15/e, pp 2515–2517.)* The disease process described is myasthenia gravis, a neuromuscular disease marked by muscle weakness and fatigability. Myasthenia gravis results from a reduction in the number of junctional acetylcholine receptors as a result of autoantibodies. Antibodies cross-link these receptors, causing a facilitation of endocytosis and degradation in lysosomes. A decreased number of available acetylcholine receptors results in decreased efficiency of neuromuscular transmission. Successive nerve impulses result in the activation of fewer muscle fibers and produce fatigue. Myasthenia presents with weakness and fatigability, particularly of cranial muscles, causing diplopia, ptosis, nasal speech, and dysarthria. Asymmetric limb weakness also occurs.

363. The answer is b. *(Braunwald, 15/e, p 2519.)* Ten percent of myasthenia patients have thymic tumors. Surgical removal of all thymomas is necessary because of local tumor spread. Even in the absence of tumor, 85% of patients clinically improve after thymectomy. It is now consensus that thymectomy be performed in all patients with generalized MG who are between puberty and age 55. Sarcoidosis causes peripheral neuropathy and aseptic meningitis, but not a myasthenia syndrome. Small cell carcinoma is associated with Lambert-Eaton syndrome, a paraneoplastic syndrome similar to myasthenia. In Lambert-Eaton syndrome, an autoimmune response results in anti–calcium channel antibodies A chest x-ray would be sufficient to screen for malignancy or infection.

364–366. The answers are 364-b, 365-a, 366-c. *(Braunwald, 15/e, pp 2274, 2397, 2399.)* A movement disorder in itself in a young person suggests Wilson's disease. This is an autosomal recessive disorder in which a deficiency in the copper-binding protein ceruloplasmin results in copper deposition in tissue. Copper deposition in the basal ganglia causes tremor and rigidity. Copper deposition in the eye produces the Kayser-Fleischer ring. Deposition in the liver causes cirrhosis and hepatitis.

The diagnosis of Parkinson's is based on resting tremor, cogwheel rigidity, and bradykinesia. Tremor is low-frequency, occurs at rest, and is pill rolling, with abduction-adduction of the thumb. Bradykinesia is usually a most striking feature. Micrographia (small handwriting) is also characteristic. Posture is often stooped with a shuffling gait and easy loss of balance.

Huntington's chorea is suspected in association with dementia and rapid, nonrhythmic movements. The disease is autosomal dominant and presents in the third or fourth decade of life. There are often slow, writhing movements called athetosis.

367. The answer is c. *(Braunwald, 15/e, pp 2423, 2430, 2507.)* This patient presents with an acute symmetrical polyneuropathy characteristic of Guillain-Barré syndrome. This is a demyelinating polyneuropathy that is often preceded by a viral illness. Characteristically, there is little sensory involvement, and about 30% of patients require ventilatory assistance. Dermatomyositis usually presents insidiously with proximal muscle weakness. Myasthenia gravis also presents insidiously with muscle weakness worsened by repetitive use. Diplopia, ptosis, and facial weakness are common first complaints. Multiple sclerosis causes demyelinating lesions disseminated in time and space and would not occur in this acute, symmetrical manner. Diabetes mellitus can cause a variety of neuropathies, but would not be rapidly progressive as in this patient.

368. The answer is a. (*Braunwald, 15/e, p 2509.*) Guillain-Barré syndrome is characterized by an elevated CSF protein with few if any white blood cells. EMG would show a demyelinating process with nonuniform slowing and conduction block. Arterial blood gases would show a respiratory acidosis secondary to hypoventilation. CPK levels should be normal, as there is no involvement of muscle in this disease process. Research laboratories show antiganglioside antibodies in as high as 50% of patients with Guillain-Barré syndrome.

369–372. The answers are 369-a, 370-d, 371-b, 372-e. (*Braunwald, 15/e, pp 2391–2398.*) The 80-year-old patient with progressive, steady memory loss and cognitive dysfunction over 2 years has not been found to have a reversible cause of dementia by standard workup. The great majority of such patients have senile dementia of the Alzheimer type. At present, there is no definitive method of premortem diagnosis, but characteristic histologic findings of neurofibrillary tangles and neuritic plaques would be noted at autopsy.

The 60-year-old woman has developed an acute clouding of consciousness and an acute confusional state described as delirium. This may occur in association with infection, drug effect, acute illness, or change in environment.

The 70-year-old with hypertension and previous stroke is most likely to have a multi-infarct dementia. This is a progressive stepwise deterioration, usually the result of recurrent bilateral cerebral infarcts. Focal findings are common, including hemiparesis, extensor plantar responses, and pseudobulbar palsy.

The patient with rapidly progressive dementia and myoclonus must be evaluated for Creutzfeldt-Jakob disease. This is a transmissible neurodegenerative dementia that shows a typical EEG pattern of periodic, bilaterally synchronous sharp wave complexes.

373–375. The answers are 373-a, 374-b, 375-d. *(Gantz, 4/e, pp 151–157.)* Fever and stiff neck with a positive quellung reaction on CSF prove the diagnosis of pneumococcal meningitis. The CSF of a patient with bacterial meningitis will show thousands of white blood cells, with more than 90% being polymorphonuclear leukocytes. The protein is always elevated, and glucose is usually lower than normal.

The patient on high-dose corticosteroids with a CSF with a positive india ink stain has cryptococcal meningitis. Cryptococcal meningitis patients usually have a lymphocytic meningitis also, with an elevated CSF protein and low CSF sugar.

The patient with focal findings and a history of dental abscess has a brain abscess. Lumbar puncture is contraindicated in the disease, but would usually show only a small number of white blood cells, if any, and a high protein and elevated CSF pressure.

376–378. The answers are 376-a, 377-b, 378-d. *(Braunwald, 15/e, pp 70–78, 1963, 2307–2310.)* Tension headaches are the leading cause of chronic headaches, and 90% are bilateral. Headaches are described as dull, constricting, and bandlike. Associated tenderness may be present.

Cluster headaches such as migraine and temporal arteritis are unilateral headaches. Cluster headaches differ from migraines in that they are nonthrobbing and are more common in men.

Temporal arteritis may cause scalp tenderness localized to the involved vessel. It is primarily a disease of the elderly. Blindness caused by occlusion of the ophthalmic artery is the feared complication.

379. The answer is a. *(Braunwald, 15/e, pp 2524–2528.)* Polymyositis is an acquired myopathy characterized by subacute symmetrical weakness of proximal limb and trunk muscles that progresses over several weeks or months. When a characteristic skin rash occurs, the disease is known as dermatomyositis. In addition to progressive proximal limb weakness, the patient often presents with dysphagia and neck muscle weakness. Up to half of cases with polymyositis-dermatomyositis may have, in addition, features of connective tissue diseases (rheumatoid arthritis, lupus erythematosus, scleroderma, Sjögren syndrome). Laboratory findings include an elevated serum CK level, an EMG showing myopathic potentials with fibrillations, and a muscle biopsy showing necrotic muscle fibers and inflammatory infiltrates. Polymyositis is clinically distinguished from the muscular dystrophies by its less prolonged course and lack of family history. It is distinguished from myasthenia gravis by its lack of ocular muscle involvement, absence of variability in strength over hours or days, and lack of response to cholinesterase inhibitor drugs.

380. The answer is d. (*Braunwald, 15/e, pp 2376–2378.*) This patient has weakness of the left face and the contralateral (right) arm and leg, commonly called a crossed hemiplegia. Such crossed syndromes are characteristic of brainstem lesions. In this case, the lesion is an infarct localized to the left inferior pons caused by occlusion of a branch of the basilar artery. The infarct has damaged the left sixth and seventh cranial nerves or nuclei in the left pons with resultant diplopia on left lateral gaze and left facial weakness. Also damaged in the left pons is the left corticospinal tract, proximal to its decussation in the medulla; this damage causes weakness in the right arm and leg. This classic presentation is called the Millard-Gubler syndrome.

381. The answer is a. (*Braunwald, 15/e, pp 76, 78, 172, 2390.*) The differential diagnosis of headaches associated with neurological or visual dysfunction is important because it encompasses a variety of disorders, some quite serious and others relatively benign. Classic (or neurological) migraine is generally a familial disorder that begins in childhood or early adult life. Typically, the onset of an episode is marked by the progression of a neurological disturbance over 5 to 15 min, followed by a unilateral (or occasionally bilateral) throbbing headache for several hours up to a day. The most common neurological disturbance involves formed or unformed flashes of light that impair vision in one of the visual fields (scintillating scotoma). Other possible neurological symptoms include numbness and tingling of the unilateral face, lips, and hand; weakness of an arm or leg; mild aphasia; and mental confusion. The transience of the neurological symptoms distinguishes migraine from other, more serious conditions that cause headaches. Persistence of a visual field defect, speech disturbance, or mild hemiparesis suggests a focal lesion (e.g., arteriovenous malformation with hemorrhage or infarct). In the case of persistent ataxia, limb incoordination, and nausea, one should consider a posterior fossa (possibly cerebellar) mass lesion.

Monocular visual loss in an elderly patient with throbbing headaches should initiate a search for cranial (temporal) arteritis. This should include a sedimentation rate (usually elevated) and a temporal artery biopsy (which would show a giant cell arteritis). Fifty percent of these patients have the generalized muscle aches seen with polymyalgia rheumatica. Unilateral orbital or retroorbital headaches that occur nightly for a period of 2 to 8 weeks are characteristic of cluster headaches. These headaches are often associated with ipsilateral injection of the conjunctivum, nasal stuffiness, rhinorrhea, and, less commonly, miosis, ptosis, and cheek edema. Although both migraine and cluster headaches may respond to treatment with ergotamine, they are generally considered to be distinct entities.

382. The answer is b. *(Braunwald, 15/e, pp 2400–2402.)* Parkinson's disease (PD) is marked by depletion of dopamine-rich cells in the substantia nigra. The resulting decrease in striatal dopamine is the basis for the classic symptoms of rigidity, bradykinesia, and tremor. By far the most widely used treatment for PD has been levodopa. Levodopa is converted to dopamine in the substantia nigra and then transported to the striatum, where it stimulates dopamine receptors. This is the basis for the drug's clinical effect on PD. Levodopa is usually administered with carbidopa (a decarboxylase inhibitor) in one pill (Sinemet), which prevents levodopa's destruction in the blood and allows it to be given at a dose that is lower and less likely to cause nausea and vomiting. The major problems with levodopa have been (1) significant limb and facial dyskinesias in most patients on chronic therapy and (2) the fact that levodopa treats PD only symptomatically, and the disease process of neuronal loss in the substantia nigra continues despite drug treatment. Other drugs can be used in the treatment of PD. Anticholinergic agents, such as trihexyphenidyl (Artane) and benztropine mesylate (Cogentin), work by restoring the balance between striatal dopamine and acetylcholine. They can have significant anticholinergic effects on the CNS, including confusional states and hallucinations. Bromocriptine and pergolide are dopamine agonists that work directly by stimulating dopamine receptors in the striatum; side effects of these drugs are similar to those of levodopa. Selegiline (Eldepryl) is a selective monoamine oxidase-B (MAO-B) inhibitor that blocks the breakdown of intracerebral dopamine.

383–386. The answers are 383-b, 384-a, 385-b, 386-d. *(Braunwald, 15/e, pp 2356–2366.)* Typical absence, or petit mal, seizure is the most characteristic epilepsy of childhood, with onset usually between age 4 and the early teens. Attacks, which may occur as frequently as several hundred times a day, consist of sudden interruptions of consciousness. The child stares, stops talking or responding, often displays eye fluttering, and commonly shows automatisms such as lip smacking and fumbling movements of the fingers. Attacks end in 2 to 10 seconds with the patient fully alert and able to resume activities. The characteristic EEG abnormality associated with attacks is three-per-second spike-and-wave activity.

Complex partial seizures, also known as psychomotor seizures, are characterized by complex auras with psychic experiences and periods of impaired consciousness with altered motor behavior. Common psychic experiences include illusions, visual or auditory hallucinations, feelings of familiarity (déjà vu) or strangeness (jamais vu), and fear or anxiety. Motor components include automatisms (e.g., lip smacking) and so-called automatic behavior (walking around in a daze, undressing in public). The brain lesion is usually in the temporal lobe, less commonly in the frontal lobe, and is often manifest as a focal epileptiform abnormality on EEG. Postictal confusion or drowsiness is the rule.

Simple partial seizures cause focal motor, sensory, or psychic symptoms without loss of consciousness.

Atonic seizures are marked by loss of postural tone. Brief loss of consciousness can occur, but there is no postictal confusion.

387–390. The answers are 387-a, 388-c, 389-b, 390-e. (*Braunwald, 15/e, pp 170, 357, 2372, 2376–2377.*) Sudden, painless monocular blindness is a sign of carotid disease. The symptom is also called amaurosis fugax. The patient may describe a shade dropping in front of the eye or describe vision like looking through ground glass. If a thrombus propagates up the carotid to the middle cerebral artery, then symptoms seen in middle cerebral artery occlusion or embolization (hemiparesis with sensory symptoms, aphasia depending on hemispheric dominance) will also occur.

Midbasilar artery disease produces weakness and sensory loss with diplopia, loss of facial sensation or movement, and ataxia. Branches of the basilar artery supply the base of the pons and superior cerebellum. The symptoms described suggest disease in the posterior circulation, which includes paired vertebral arteries, the basilar artery, and the paired posterior cerebral arteries. The basilar artery divides into two posterior cerebral arteries that provide branches to the cerebellum, medulla, pons, midbrain, thalamus, and temporal and occipital lobes. A midbasilar artery occlusion could cause ataxia of limbs by involving pontine nuclei; paralysis of the face, arm, and leg by involving corticospinal tracts; and impairment of facial sensation by involvement of fifth nerve nucleus.

Occlusion of the entire middle cerebral artery results in contralateral hemiplegia, hemianesthesia, and homonymous hemianopsia. When the dominant hemisphere is involved, aphasia is present. When the nondominant hemisphere is involved, apraxia and neglect are produced. When only a penetrating branch of the middle cerebral artery is affected, the syndrome of pure motor hemiplegia is produced, as the infarct involves only the posterior limb of the internal capsule, involving only motor fibers to the face, arm, and leg (lacunar infarct).

Dermatology

Questions

DIRECTIONS: Each item below contains a question or incomplete statement followed by suggested responses. Select the **one best** response to each question.

391. A 20-year-old woman complains of skin problems and is noted to have erythematous papules on her face with blackheads (open comedones) and whiteheads (closed comedones). She has also had cystic lesions. She is prescribed a topical tretinoin (Retin-A), but without a totally acceptable result. Which of the following is correct?

a. Intralesional triamcinolone should be avoided due to its systemic effects
b. Systemically administered isotretinoin therapy cannot be considered unless concomitant contraceptive therapy is provided
c. Antimicrobial therapy is of no value since bacteria are not part of the pathogenesis of the process
d. Isotretinoin is without important side effects as long as it is not used in sexually active women

392. A 22-year-old male presents with a 6-month history of a red, nonpruritic rash over the trunk, scalp, elbows, and knees. These eruptions are more likely to occur during stressful periods and have occurred at sites of skin injury. On exam, sharply demarcated plaques are seen with a thick scale (see photo). Which of the following statements is correct?

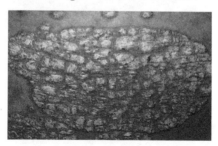

a. The lesions are contagious and contact should be carefully avoided
b. The patient is allergic to metals
c. The clinical description is most consistent with psoriasis
d. The rash is unrelated to stress

393. A 25-year-old complains of fever and myalgias for 5 days and now has developed a macular rash over his palms and soles with some petechial lesions. The patient recently returned from a summer camping trip in the Great Smoky Mountains. The most likely cause of the rash is

a. Contact dermatitis
b. Sexual exposure
c. Tick exposure
d. Contaminated stream

394. A 17-year-old female presents with a pruritic rash localized to the wrist. Papules and vesicles are noted in a bandlike pattern, with slight oozing from some lesions. The most likely cause of the rash is

a. Herpes simplex
b. Shingles
c. Contact dermatitis
d. Seborrheic dermatitis

Items 395–396

395. A 35-year-old woman develops an itchy rash over her back, legs, and trunk several hours after swimming in a lake. Erythematous, edematous papules are noted. The wheals vary in size. There are no mucosal lesions and no swelling of the lips (see photo). The most likely diagnosis is

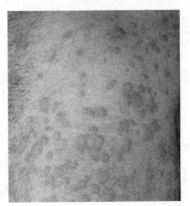

a. Urticaria
b. Folliculitis
c. Erythema multiforme
d. Erythema chronicum migrans

396. The treatment of choice for this patient is

a. Epinephrine
b. Intravenous glucocorticoids
c. Antihistamines and avoidance of offending agent
d. Aspirin

397. A 30-year-old black female has had a history of cough, and a chest x-ray shows bilateral hilar lymphadenopathy. A biopsy shows noncaseating granuloma. The skin lesion most consistent with the patient's diagnosis is

a. Seborrheic keratosis
b. Asymmetric pigmented lesion with irregular border
c. Erythema nodosum
d. Umbilicated, dome-shaped yellow papules

Items 398–399

398. An elderly homeless male is evaluated for anemia. On exam, he has purpura and ecchymoses of the legs. Perifollicular papules and perifollicular hemorrhages are also noted. There is swelling and bleeding of gums around the patient's teeth as well as tenderness around a hematoma of the calf. The most likely diagnosis is

a. Elder abuse
b. Scurvy
c. Pellagra
d. Beriberi

399. The best approach to the management of this patient is

a. Obtain platelet ascorbic acid level and give ascorbic acid while in hospital
b. Discharge with dietary consult
c. Give folic acid
d. Obtain plasma tryptophan

400. A 50-year-old woman develops pink macules and papules on her hands and forearms in association with a sore throat. The lesions are target-like, with the centers a dusky violet (see photo). A diagnosis of erythema multiforme is made. The most important information obtained from this patient's history is

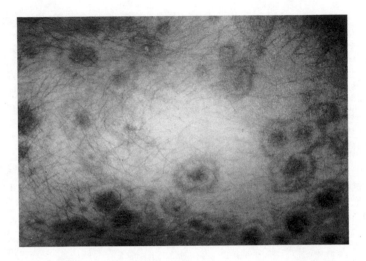

a. The patient has been using tampons
b. The patient is taking phenytoin
c. The patient has never had measles
d. No other family members have a sore throat

401. A 25-year-old female with blonde hair and fair complexion complains of a mole on her upper back. The lesion is 6 mm in diameter, darkly pigmented, and asymmetric, with a very irregular border (see photo). The next step in management is

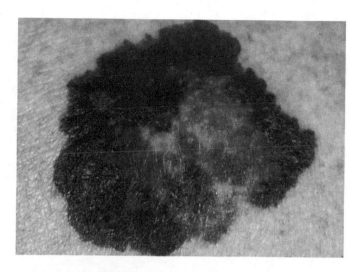

a. Tell the patient to avoid sunlight
b. Follow the lesion for any evidence of growth
c. Obtain metastatic workup
d. Obtain full-thickness excisional biopsy
e. Obtain shave biopsy

402. A 39-year-old male with a prior history of myocardial infarction complains of yellow bumps on his elbows and buttocks. Yellow-colored cutaneous plaques are noted in those areas. The lesions occur in crops and have a surrounding reddish halo. The next step in evaluation of this patient is

a. Biopsy of skin lesions
b. Lipid profile
c. Uric acid levels
d. Chest x-ray to evaluate for sarcoidosis

403. A 15-year-old girl complains of a low-grade fever, malaise, conjunctivitis, coryza, and cough. After this prodromal phase, a rash of discrete pink macules begins on her face and extends to her hands and feet. She is also noted to have small red spots on her palate. The cause of her rash is

a. Toxic shock syndrome
b. Gonococcal bacteremia
c. Reiter syndrome
d. Rubeola (measles)
e. Rubella (German measles)

404. A 17-year-old girl noted a 2-cm annular pink, scaly lesion on her thigh. In the next 2 weeks she developed several smaller oval pink lesions with a fine collarette of scale. They seem to run in the body folds and mainly involve the trunk, although a few are on the upper arms and thighs. There is no adenopathy and no oral lesions. The most likely diagnosis is

a. Tinea versicolor
b. Psoriasis
c. Lichen planus
d. Pityriasis rosea
e. Secondary syphilis

405. A 45-year-old man with Parkinson's disease has macular areas of erythema and scaling behind the ears and on the scalp, eyebrows, glabella, nasolabial folds, and central chest. The diagnosis is

a. Tinea versicolor
b. Psoriasis
c. Seborrheic dermatitis
d. Atopic dermatitis
e. Dermatophyte infection

406. A 20-year-old white man notes an uneven tan on his upper back and chest. On examination, he has many circular, lighter macules with a barely visible scale that coalesce into larger areas. The best test procedure to establish the diagnosis is

a. Punch biopsy
b. Potassium hydroxide (KOH) microscopic examination
c. Dermatophyte test medium (DTM) culture for fungus
d. Serological test for syphilis
e. Tzanck smear

407. A 33-year-old fair-skinned woman has telangiectasias of the cheeks and nose along with red papules and occasional pustules. She also appears to have a conjunctivitis because of dilated scleral vessels. She reports frequent flushing and blushing. Drinking red wine produces a severe flushing of the face. There is a family history of this condition. The diagnosis is

a. Carcinoid syndrome
b. Porphyria cutanea tarda
c. Lupus vulgaris
d. Acne rosacea
e. Seborrheic dermatitis

408. A 22-year-old man from New Jersey suddenly develops a pruritic vesicular rash on his arms, hands, and face. There are linear areas of blisters. The rash appears to be spreading for 2 days. Four days previously he was clearing out a wooded area in his yard. The diagnosis is

a. Chickenpox
b. Lyme disease
c. Blister beetle bites
d. Poison ivy
e. Photosensitivity reaction

409. A 25-year-old postal worker presents with a pruritic, nonpainful skin lesion on the dorsum of his hand. It began looking like an insect bite but expanded over several days. On exam, the lesion has a black, necrotic center and is associated with swelling. The patient does not appear to be systemically ill, and vital signs are normal. Which of the following is correct?

a. The lesion is ecthyma gangrenosum, and blood cultures will be positive for *Pseudomonas aeruginosa*
b. A skin biopsy should be performed and Gram stain examined for gram-positive rods
c. The patient has been bitten by *Loxosceles reclusa,* the brown recluse spider
d. The patient has the bubo of plague

410. A 25-year-old who has been living in Washington, DC presents with a diffuse vesicular rash over his face and trunk. He also has fever. He has no history of chickenpox and has not received the chickenpox vaccine. Which of the following information obtained from history and physical exam suggests that the patient has chickenpox and not smallpox?

a. There are vesicular lesions on the palms and soles
b. All lesions are at the same stage of development
c. The patient experienced high fever several days prior to the rash
d. The rash is more dense over the face than the trunk
e. None of the above

411. A 21-year-old health care worker has been vaccinated for smallpox. After 2 weeks, the site of inoculation fails to heal and the lesion progresses in size with central necrosis and dark eschars. There is little surrounding inflammatory reaction and no pustular lesions. Which of the following is correct?

a. This is a smallpox vaccine complication called vaccinia necrosum; the treatment of choice is vaccinia immune globulin
b. The most likely diagnosis is erythema multiforme
c. The patient is likely to have underlying eczema
d. No evaluation for underlying disease process is necessary

Dermatology

Answers

391. The answer is b. (*Stobo, 23/e, p 984.*) Isotretinoin has a high potential for teratogenicity and should not be used in women in their childbearing years unless contraception is being practiced. The drug also causes hypertriglyceridemia and drying of mucous membranes. It should be reserved for severe cystic acne. Intralesional triamcinolone is effective for occasional cystic lesions and does not cause systemic side effects. Antimicrobial therapy is of value, in part due to its suppressive effect on *Propionibacterium acnes*. Oral tetracyclines and topical metronidazole are most commonly used.

392. The answer is c. (*Braunwald, 15/e, p 311.*) The rash described is classic for psoriasis, an extremely common chronic inflammatory skin disorder. Its characteristic features include sharply bordered, often round papules or plaques with silver scale, usually located on the knees, elbows, and scalp. Stress, certain medications such as lithium, and skin injury commonly exacerbate the disease. The distribution of the described rash would make contact dermatitis unlikely. Psoriasis is not contagious and is not spread by contact. In the differential of psoriasis is lichen planus (polygonal pruritic purple papules with lacy mucous membrane lesions), pityriasis rosea (herald patch occurs first, on trunk in Christmas tree pattern), and dermatophytes (usually less well demarcated, affecting skin, hair, and nails).

393. The answer is c. (*Braunwald, 15/e, p 1065.*) The rash described is most consistent with Rocky Mountain spotted fever, for which a tick is the intermediate vector. Secondary syphilis could present with a macular rash in the same distribution, but the associated symptoms would be atypical. Contact dermatitis would not cause petechial lesions.

394. The answer is c. (*Braunwald, 15/e, p 309.*) Contact dermatitis causes pruritic plaques or vesicles localized to an area of contact. In this case, a bracelet or wristband would be the inciting agent. The dermatitis may have vesicles with weeping lesions. The process is related to direct irritation of the skin from a chemical or physical irritant. It may also be immune-mediated. Zoster would be painful and occur in a dermatomal distribution. Herpes simplex produces grouped vesicles, but they are painful and also unlikely to occur around the wrist. Seborrheic dermatitis presents as red, scaly lesions over a circular area with lesions developing in the nasolabial folds, scalp, and retroauricular areas.

395. The answer is a. *(Braunwald, 15/e, pp 318, 323, 822, 1061, 1917–1918.)* Urticaria, or hives, is a common dermatologic problem characterized by pruritic, edematous papules and plaques that vary in size and come and go, often within hours. Mast cells may be stimulated by heat, cold, pressure, water, or exercise. Immunologic mechanisms can also cause mast cell degranulation. Folliculitis caused by *Pseudomonas aeruginosa* can cause a rash, often after exposure to hot tubs. The lesions would not be as diffuse, with a line of demarcation depending on the water level. These lesions are pustular and occur 8 to 48 h after soaking. Erythema multiforme produces target-like lesions and oral blisters often secondary to medications. Erythema chronicum migrans usually presents with a large, solitary annular lesion.

396. The answer is c. *(Braunwald, 15/e, pp 1917–1918.)* Avoidance of the offending agent, when it is identifiable, is most important in management of urticaria. Oral antihistamines provide symptomatic relief. Agents such as aspirin or alcohol, which aggravate cutaneous vasodilation, are contraindicated. Glucocorticoids play a minimal role in management of urticaria unless the process is severe and unremitting. Epinephrine plays no role in treatment unless there is concomitant anaphylaxis.

397. The answer is c. *(Braunwald, 15/e, pp 1970–1972.)* Erythema nodosum is a hypersensitivity reaction associated with this patient's sarcoidosis. Keratoses, melanoma (as described in option b), and molluscum contagiosum (as described in option d) are not associated with sarcoidosis.

398. The answer is b. *(Braunwald, 15/e, p 464.)* The signs and symptoms described are most consistent with scurvy (vitamin C deficiency). This syndrome can occur in older patients who are poorly nourished. Perifollicular papules develop when hairs become fragmented and buried in the follicle. Capillary fragility occurs, and bleeding into soft tissue is common. Pellagra (vitamin B_3 deficiency) causes a dermatitis that is symmetrical and related to photosensitivity. Beriberi (vitamin B_1 deficiency) does not typically cause a rash, but presents with high-output cardiac failure, peripheral neuropathy, and Wernicke's encephalopathy. The perifollicular nature of the bleeding described in this patient does not suggest a traumatic etiology.

399. The answer is a. *(Braunwald, 15/e, p 464.)* Platelet ascorbic acid levels are the best approach to documenting this deficiency. Ascorbic acid 100 mg should be given three to five times per day until 4 g have been given. Scurvy is potentially fatal, and the patient should not be discharged until supplementation is guaranteed. Folic acid levels should be checked concomitantly to identify folate deficiency and folate should be given if necessary. Tryptophan levels are used in evaluating for pellagra.

400. The answer is b. *(Braunwald, 15/e, pp 337–339.)* Erythema multiforme is often caused by drugs. It is most important to identify the offending agent. Phenytoin can induce erythema multiforme, so this information is critical. Sulfa drugs, barbiturates, and penicillin can also be causes. The rash, with its target lesions, should not be confused with toxic shock or measles. The sore throat is likely to be a symptom from the process itself, suggesting involvement of the oral mucosa.

401. The answer is d. *(Braunwald, 15/e, pp 554–557.)* The lesion has characteristics of melanoma (pigmentation, asymmetry, irregular border), and a full-thickness excisional biopsy is required. Shave biopsy of a suspected melanoma is always contraindicated. Diagnosis is urgent; the lesion cannot be observed over time. Once the diagnosis of melanoma is made, the tumor must then be staged to determine prognosis and treatment.

402. The answer is b. *(Braunwald, 15/e, pp 326–328.)* The description and location of these lesions are suggestive of xanthoma. Eruptive xanthomas occur primarily on extensor surfaces and are associated with elevated triglycerides. Tophaceous gout can result in deposits of monosodium urate, usually in the skin around joints of the hands and feet, that may also be yellow in color. The cutaneous lesions of sarcoidosis are more red-brown in color, appearing as waxy papules, usually on the face. Treatment of hypertriglyceridemia usually results in resolution of lesions. Biopsy of xanthoma would show lipid-containing macrophages, but is usually not necessary for diagnosis.

403. The answer is d. *(Freedberg, 5/e, pp 2399–2400.)* The patient presents with the classic picture of measles. Coryza, conjunctivitis, cough, and fever characterize the measles prodrome. The pathognomonic Koplik spots (pinpoint elevations connected by a network of minute vessels on the soft palate) usually precede onset of the rash by 24 to 48 h and may remain for 2 or 3 days. After the prodrome of 1 to 7 days, the discrete red macules and papules begin behind the ears and spread to the face and trunk, and then distally over the extremities. Toxic shock syndrome produces a diffuse, macular, sunburn-like rash with mucosal hyperemia. Gonococcal bacteremia is more likely to cause nodular skin lesions. In rubella, a maculopapular rash is associated with petechial lesions of the soft palate. Cervical lymphadenopathy is a prominent feature.

404. The answer is d. *(Freedberg, 5/e, pp 541–545.)* The description of this papulosquamous disease is that of a classic case of pityriasis rosea. This disease occurs in about 10% of the population. It is usually seen in young adults on the trunk and proximal extremities. There is a rare inverse form that occurs in the distal extremities and occasionally the face. Pityriasis rosea is usually asymptomatic, although some patients have an early, mild viral prodrome (malaise and low-grade fever), and itching may be significant. Drug eruptions, fungal infections, and secondary syphilis are often confused with this disease. Fungal infections are rarely as widespread and sudden in onset; potassium hydroxide (KOH) preparation will be positive. Syphilis usually is characterized by adenopathy, oral patches, and lesions on the palms and soles (a VDRL test will be strongly positive at this stage). Psoriasis, with its thick, scaly red plaques on extensor surfaces, should not cause confusion. A rare condition called guttate parapsoriasis should be suspected if the rash lasts more than 2 months, since pityriasis rosea usually clears spontaneously in 6 weeks.

405. The answer is c. *(Freedberg, 5/e, pp 1482–1487.)* The patient has the typical areas of involvement of seborrheic dermatitis. This common dermatitis appears to be worse in many neurological diseases. It is also very common and severe in patients with AIDS. In general, symptoms are worse in the winter. *Pityrosporum ovale* appears to play a role in seborrheic dermatitis and dandruff, and the symptoms improve with the use of certain antifungal preparations (e.g., ketoconazole) that decrease this yeast. Mild topical steroids also produce an excellent clinical response.

406. The answer is b. *(Freedberg, 5/e, pp 36–37, 2368–2370.)* The diagnosis is tinea versicolor, which can be easily confirmed by a KOH microscopic examination. Routine fungal cultures will not grow this yeast. A Wood's light examination will often show a green fluorescence, but it may be negative if the patient has recently showered. A Tzanck smear is used on vesicles to detect herpes infection. A punch biopsy would show the fungus, but is unnecessary, and the fungus might be missed unless special stains are performed.

407. The answer is d. *(Freedberg, 5/e, pp 785–787.)* Rosacea is a common problem in middle-aged, fair-skinned people. Sun damage appears to play an important role. Stress, alcohol, and heat cause flushing. Men may develop rhinophyma (connective tissue overgrowth, particularly of the nose). Low-dose oral tetracycline, erythromycin, and metronidazole control the symptoms. Topical erythromycin and metronidazole also work well.

408. The answer is d. *(Freeberg, 5/e, pp 1609–1613.)* In an allergic person, poison ivy *(Rhus)* dermatitis begins 24 to 48 h after exposure to the oil from the plant. Linear blisters are an important clue to the diagnosis. It is an allergic contact dermatitis. The sensitizing antigen is urushiol, an oleoresin. The oleoresin may adhere to clothes, pets, or other articles, producing a delayed exposure.

409. The answer is b. *(Braunwald, 15/e, pp 763, 914.)* The possibility of cutaneous anthrax in this postal worker is the most important consideration in the era of bioterrorism concern. The lesion described would be characteristic of cutaneous anthrax—beginning as a small papule that is painless and progressing to a black, necrotic lesion over several days. A skin biopsy would show the very characteristic gram-positive rods of anthrax. Cutaneous anthrax has been shown to occur in postal workers who have handled letters that contained anthrax spores, and can also occur in those who handle infected animals or their wool or hides. Ecthyma gangrenosum also produces a black, necrotic skin lesion. These lesions occur in patients who are bacteremic and systemically ill from *P. aeruginosa.* The brown recluse spider's bite can also produce a necrotic ulcer that is black. The bite is painful and usually spreads rapidly. The bubo of plague produces a tender lymphadenitis. It too occurs in a patient who is systemically ill.

410. The answer is e. (Henderson) Although there have been no cases of smallpox in the world since 1977, the threat of bioterrorism has forced physicians to be vigilant about the disease's reemergence. It will be important for students and physicians to recognize the distinguishing characteristics of smallpox versus chickenpox. All of the history and physical findings in this case suggest smallpox. Lesions are more likely to occur on palms and soles in smallpox. In chickenpox, lesions are more concentrated on the trunk, whereas in smallpox they are likely to be more concentrated on the face. In smallpox, lesions are characteristically in the same stage of development. In chickenpox, lesions are more superficial, come out in crops, and are in many different stages of development. In smallpox, patients are much more systemically ill, and give a history of fever and prostration prior to the development of the rash. In chickenpox, fever usually occurs at the time of the appearance of the rash.

411. The answer is a. (Mandell, 5/e, p 1554.) The complication of smallpox vaccine described is called vaccinia necrosum or progressive vaccinia. In this disease process, the normal response to vaccination is impaired. The site of the live vaccinia virus inoculation continues to enlarge and fails to heal. As it progresses in size, central necrosis usually occurs. There is little inflammatory reaction. It is usually easily distinguishable from bacterial superinfection. Administration of vaccinia immune globulin is considered the treatment of choice. This immune globulin may be in short supply. Erythema multiforme does occur as an allergic reaction to the vaccine. It is a diffuse erythematous rash with bull's-eye lesions. In patients with eczema, typical vaccinia-type lesions can occur in the areas of active eczema. This process, called eczema vaccinatum, can also be very serious, and patients with eczema should not receive the smallpox vaccine if it can be avoided. In a patient with vaccinia necrosum, it is important to consider underlying immunodeficiency disease such as HIV or other immunodeficiency disease.

General Medicine and Prevention

Questions

DIRECTIONS: Each item below contains a question or incomplete statement followed by suggested responses. Select the **one best** response to each question.

412. A 38-year-old patient presents to the emergency room with a minor injury and is found to have a blood pressure of 145/95. The best approach to follow-up of this patient's blood pressure is

a. Full diagnostic evaluation immediately
b. Full diagnostic evaluation within 1 month
c. Confirm another high blood pressure reading within 2 months and provide advice on lifestyle modifications
d. Recheck blood pressure within 1 year and provide advice on lifestyle modifications
e. Recheck blood pressure in 2 years

413. You are evaluating a newly diagnosed middle-aged adult with diabetes. Which of the following is least likely to be of value in diabetic management?

a. Blood pressure check
b. Eye exam
c. Foot exam
d. Hemoglobin A_{1c}
e. Lipid profile
f. Liver function tests
g. Urine microalbumin level

414. Which of the following represents the currently recommended goal for blood pressure control in a diabetic?

a. Less than 160/90
b. Less than 145/95
c. Less than 140/90
d. Less than 130/85
e. Less than 120/70

Items 415–416

415. A 60-year-old white male just moved to town and needs to establish care for coronary artery disease. He had a heart attack last year, but gradually eliminated several prescription medications (he does not recall the names) that he was on at the time of hospital discharge. However, he has been very conscientious about low-fat, low-cholesterol eating habits. Past history is negative for hypertension, diabetes, or smoking. The lipid profile you obtain shows the following:

Total cholesterol: 210 mg/dL
Triglycerides: 190
HDL: 52
LDL (calculated): 120

To optimally treat his lipid status, you suggest which of the following?

a. Continue dietary efforts
b. Add an HMG-CoA reductase inhibitor (statin drug)
c. Add a fibric acid derivative such as gemfibrozil
d. Review his previous medications and resume an angiotensin converting enzyme inhibitor

416. In the preceding patient, for secondary prevention of further myocardial infarction, the patient should be placed on (in addition to aspirin)

a. Alpha blocker therapy
b. Beta blocker therapy
c. Calcium channel blocker therapy
d. Nitrates

Items 417–418

417. A 50-year-old white male who comes for general checkup is a healthy nonsmoker, free of hypertension, diabetes, or cardiac disease; however, his 53-year-old brother had coronary artery bypass surgery this year. You order a fasting lipid profile. Which of the following LDL target levels do you have in mind?

a. Less than 160 mg/dL
b. Less than 130 mg/dL
c. Less than 100 mg/dL
d. None specifically required based on current risks

418. In the preceding patient, if the good HDL cholesterol is found to be low, an important recommendation for trying to elevate this would be

a. Aspirin, one tablet each day
b. Dehydroepiandrosterone (DHEA)
c. Vitamin E, 400 U each day
d. Folic acid plus pyridoxine (vitamin B_6)
e. Exercise

419. A 32-year-old diabetic female who takes an estrogen-containing oral contraceptive and drinks three beers per day is found to have a triglyceride level greater than 1000 mg/dL. She is at risk for which of the following complications?

a. Acute pancreatitis
b. Sudden cardiac death
c. Acute peripheral arterial occlusion
d. Acute renal insufficiency
e. Myositis

420. A 28-year-old, otherwise healthy white female on no medications presents to the ER with chest pressure, dizziness, numbness in both hands, and feeling of impending doom that began while walking in the mall. The most likely diagnosis on the differential is

a. Angina
b. Congenital heart disease
c. Gastroesophageal reflux
d. Panic disorder
e. Pulmonary embolus

421. A 45-year-old, generally healthy female on no medications comes to your office with a 10-day history of nasal congestion, sore throat, dry cough, and initial low-grade fever, all of which were nearly resolved. However, over the past 24 to 48 h she has developed a sharp chest pain, worse with deep inspiration or cough, but no dyspnea. Due to the severity of the pain, the nurse had obtained an ECG, which showed diffuse ST elevation. On physical exam, you expect the most likely finding to be

a. A loud pulmonic component of S_2
b. An S_3 gallop
c. A pericardial friction rub
d. Bilateral basilar rales
e. Elevated blood pressure >160/100

422. A 25-year-old Hispanic male PhD candidate recently traveled to rural Mexico for 1 month to gain further information for his dissertation regarding socioeconomics. While there, he took ciprofloxacin for diarrhea. However, over the 2 to 3 weeks since coming home, he has continued to have occasional loose stools plus vague abdominal discomfort and bloating. There has been no rectal bleeding. The most likely cause of this traveler's diarrhea is

a. *Campylobacter jejuni*
b. Toxigenic *Escherichia coli*
c. *Giardia lamblia*
d. *Cryptosporidium*
e. *Salmonella*
f. *Shigella*

423. A 25-year-old asymptomatic HIV-positive male comes to you for travel advice and immunizations prior to a trip to Indonesia. Which of the following is an inappropriate recommendation?

a. Give tetanus-diphtheria booster if not up to date
b. Give oral polio booster if not up to date
c. Start hepatitis B immunization series if never received
d. Give pneumococcal vaccine if never received
e. Give second MMR if only one dose previously received
f. Give malaria prophylaxis

424. In August you saw a debilitated 80-year-old female who required nursing home placement. She had had no immunizations for many years except for a pneumococcal vaccine 3 years ago when discharged from the hospital after a stay for pneumonia. Appropriate admission orders to the nursing home in August included

a. Flu shot
b. *Haemophilus influenzae* B immunization
c. Hepatitis B immunization series
d. Pneumococcal revaccination
e. Tetanus-diphtheria toxoid booster

425. An asymptomatic 50-year-old man who has smoked one pack of cigarettes per day for 30 years comes to you for a general checkup and wants "the works" for cancer screening. In fact, he hands you a list of tests he desires. Which test is inappropriate based on American Cancer Society guidelines?

a. Chest x-ray
b. Digital rectal exam
c. Flexible sigmoidoscopy
d. Prostate-specific antigen (PSA) blood test
e. Skin exam

426. An asymptomatic 35-year-old female comes to you for routine exam. She has no unusual family history of breast cancer. Based on American Cancer Society guidelines for early detection of breast cancer, this patient at standard risk should be advised to

a. Perform breast self-examination monthly
b. Obtain physician-performed breast examination yearly
c. Begin yearly mammograms
d. Obtain genetic testing via blood work as a baseline
e. Wait until age 40 to begin cancer screening

427. On presentation for yearly exam, a healthy, non–sexually active postmenopausal 60-year-old female gives a history of having had normal yearly mammograms and normal yearly Pap smears over the past 10 years, but never an endometrial tissue sample or any screening test for ovarian cancer. The most clearly indicated cancer screening evaluation on today's visit is

a. Bilateral mammogram
b. Pap smear
c. Endometrial tissue sample
d. CA 125 blood test
e. CEA level

428. You have been asked to perform a preoperative consultation on a 65-year-old male who will be undergoing transurethral resection of the prostate for urinary retention. Of the following findings, which you detect by history, physical, and lab, which is of most concern in predicting a cardiac complication in this patient undergoing noncardiac surgery?

a. Age over 60
b. History of myocardial infarction 2 years ago
c. Harsh systolic crescendo-decrescendo murmur radiating to the carotids
d. ECG and subsequent cardiac monitoring showing up to five PVCs per minute
e. Serum creatinine 2.0 mg/dL

429. A 42-year-old male is persuaded by his wife to come to you for general checkup. She hints of concern about alcohol use. Therefore, you ask the CAGE questions as an initial screen. These include which of the following?

a. Concern expressed by family
b. Previous Alcoholics Anonymous contact
c. Alcohol intake greater than two drinks per 24 h
d. Gastrointestinal symptoms
e. Use of an eye-opener
f. Presence of excess extremity shakiness

430. A 78-year-old female comes to your office with symptoms of insomnia nearly every day, fatigue, weight loss of over 5% of body weight over the past month, loss of interest in most activities, and diminished ability to concentrate. Although further testing may be necessary, based on this history the most likely diagnosis is

a. Alzheimer's dementia
b. Anemia
c. Collagen-vascular disease with CNS involvement
d. Depression
e. Hypothyroidism
f. Parkinson's disease

431. A 65-year-old female was hospitalized for pulmonary embolus and eventually discharged on warfarin (Coumadin) with a therapeutic INR. During the next 2 weeks as an outpatient, she was started back on her previous ACE inhibitor antihypertensive, given temazepam for insomnia, treated with ciprofloxacin for a urinary tract infection, started on famotidine prophylaxis for peptic ulcer disease, and told to stop the over-the-counter naproxen she was taking. Follow-up INR was too high, most likely due to

a. ACE inhibitor therapy
b. Temazepam
c. Ciprofloxacin
d. Famotidine
e. Naproxen discontinuation

432. A 20-year-old college basketball player is brought to the university urgent care clinic after developing chest pain and palpitations during practice, but no dyspnea or tachypnea. There is no unusual family history of cardiac diseases, and social history is negative for alcohol or drug use. Cardiac auscultation is unremarkable, and ECG shows only occasional PVCs. The next step in evaluation and/or management should be to

a. Obtain urine drug screen
b. Arrange treadmill stress test
c. Obtain Doppler ultrasound of deep veins of lower legs
d. Institute cardioselective beta blocker therapy
e. Institute respiratory therapy for this form of exercise-induced bronchospasm

DIRECTIONS: Each group of questions below consists of lettered options followed by a set of numbered items. For each numbered item, select the **one** lettered option with which it is **most** closely associated. Each lettered option may be used once, more than once, or not at all.

Items 433–435

The initial choice of an antihypertensive agent may depend on concomitant factors. For each of the conditions below, indicate the medication choice that would give the best additional benefit after blood pressure control.

a. Alpha blocker
b. Beta blocker
c. Calcium channel blocker
d. Angiotensin converting enzyme inhibitor
e. Centrally acting agent

433. Benign prostatic hypertrophy with urinary retention **(CHOOSE 1 MEDICATION)**

434. Diabetes with proteinuria **(CHOOSE 1 MEDICATION)**

435. Migraine headache or essential tremor **(CHOOSE 1 MEDICA-TION)**

Items 436–439

The choice of an antihypertensive agent may involve trying to avoid an adverse effect on a comorbid condition. For each of the conditions below, indicate the medication choice that needs to be avoided above all others.

a. Angiotensin converting enzyme inhibitor
b. Beta blocker, noncardioselective
c. Calcium channel blocker
d. Diuretic
e. Hydralazine

436. Acute gout **(CHOOSE 1 MEDICATION)**

437. Asthma **(CHOOSE 1 MEDICATION)**

438. Peripheral vascular disease **(CHOOSE 1 MEDICATION)**

439. Pregnancy, second and third trimester **(CHOOSE 1 MEDICATION)**

440. A 92-year-old woman with type 2 diabetes mellitus has developed cellulitis and gangrene of her left foot. She requires a lifesaving amputation, but refuses to give consent for the surgery. She has been ambulatory in her nursing home but states that she would be so dependent after surgery that life would not be worth living for her. She has no living relatives; she enjoys walks and gardening. She is competent and of clear mind. You should

a. Perform emergency surgery
b. Consult a psychiatrist
c. Request permission for surgery from a friend of the patient
d. Follow the patient's wishes

441. A 20-year-old complains of diarrhea, burning of the throat, and difficulty swallowing over 2 months. On exam, he has mild jaundice and transverse white striae of the fingernails. There is also evidence for peripheral neuropathy. The best diagnostic study is

a. Liver biopsy
b. Arsenic level
c. Antinuclear antibody
d. Endoscopy (EGD)

442. A young boy believes he was bitten by a spider while playing in his attic. Severe pain develops at the site of the bite after several hours. Bullae and erythema develop around the bite, and some skin necrosis becomes apparent. The boy is afebrile without evidence of toxicity. Which of the following is correct?

a. The boy most likely was bitten by a black widow spider
b. The boy was most likely bitten by a *Loxosceles* (brown recluse) spider
c. Antivenin is the approved method of treatment
d. The patient has necrotizing fasciitis secondary to streptococcal infection

443. A 70-year-old male with unresectable carcinoma of the lung metastatic to liver and bone has developed progressive weight loss, anorexia, and shortness of breath. The patient has executed a valid living will that prohibits the use of feeding tube in the setting of terminal illness. The patient becomes lethargic and stops eating altogether. The patient's wife of 30 years insists on enteral feeding for her husband. Since he has become unable to take in adequate nutrition, you should

a. Respect the wife's wishes as a reliable surrogate decision maker
b. Resist the placement of a feeding tube in accordance with the living will
c. Call a family conference to get broad input from others
d. Place a feeding tube until such time as the matter can be discussed with the patient

444. After being stung by a yellow jacket, a 14-year-old develops the sudden onset of hoarseness and shortness of breath. An urticarial rash is noted. The most important first step in treatment is

a. Antihistamine
b. Epinephrine
c. Venom immunotherapy
d. Corticosteroids
e. Removal of stinger

445. A 40-year-old male is found to have a uric acid level of 9 mg/dL on routine screening of blood chemistry. The patient has never had gouty arthritis, renal disease, or kidney stones. The patient has no evidence on history or physical exam of underlying chronic or malignant disease. Which of the following is correct?

a. The risk of urolithiasis requires the institution of prophylactic therapy
b. Asymptomatic hyperuricemia is associated with an increased risk of gouty arthritis, but benefits of prophylaxis do not outweigh risks in this patient
c. The presence or absence of lymphoproliferative disease does not affect the decision to use prophylaxis in hyperuricemia
d. Lowering serum uric acid will provide a direct cardiovascular benefit to the patient in lowering coronary artery disease risk

Items 446–451

For each patient, select the best course of action.

a. Begin isoniazid chemoprophylaxis
b. No prophylaxis indicated
c. Begin therapy for tuberculosis using three to four drugs
d. Begin therapy for tuberculosis using a two-drug regimen
e. Repeat PPD in 2 weeks

446. An HIV-positive patient with 5-mm PPD **(SELECT 1 COURSE OF ACTION)**

447. A 30-year-old hospital employee with 15-mm PPD; previous status unknown **(SELECT 1 COURSE OF ACTION)**

448. A 70-year-old new patient at a nursing home with 8-mm PPD **(SELECT 1 COURSE OF ACTION)**

449. A 50-year-old patient with Hodgkin's disease; 12-mm PPD, fever, abnormal chest x-ray; one sputum smear positive for acid-fast bacillus **(SELECT 1 COURSE OF ACTION)**

450. A 40-year-old with 10-mm PPD; no underlying illness; first time ever done **(SELECT 1 COURSE OF ACTION)**

451. A 60-year-old woman with negative PPD 1 year ago; now with 12-mm PPD on annual screening **(SELECT 1 COURSE OF ACTION)**

General Medicine and Prevention

Answers

412. The answer is c. (*JNC VI, p 13.*) One should neither jump to the diagnosis of hypertension too quickly nor delay follow-up too long. Most patients will require a second visit to confirm the diagnosis of essential hypertension.

413. The answer is f. (*Braunwald, 15/e, pp 2127–2129.*) All of the listed choices are very important except for liver function tests. Annual evaluation (assuming all is normal) is recommended for blood pressure check, eye exam, lipid profile, and urine microalbumin level; evaluation every 6 to 12 months is recommended for foot exam. Hemoglobin A_{1c} (or similar test) should be obtained every 6 months if stable, or quarterly if treatment changes or the patient is not achieving goals.

414. The answer is d. (*JNC VI, p 49.*) Goals for blood pressure control and lipid levels are typically more stringent in the diabetic compared to the nondiabetic. Blood pressure less than 130/85 is recommended.

415. The answer is b. (*NCEP ATP III, pp 2486–2489.*) The National Cholesterol Education Program Adult Treatment Panel III includes lowering the LDL cholesterol to less than 100 in those with known coronary heart disease (secondary prevention). If dietary efforts are in place, a statin drug will likely be required. Gemfibrozil is used primarily for hypertriglyceridemia. ACE inhibitors have no significant effect on lipids.

416. The answer is b. (*Braunwald, 15/e, pp 1399, 1405.*) Beta blockers are documented to lower the risk of myocardial reinfarction, whereas calcium channel blockers may increase the risk. ACE inhibitors are beneficial in this setting, and the data is accumulating that angiotensin II receptor blockers are as well. Despite their decades-long use in the treatment of coronary artery disease, such as for angina, nitrates are not indicated for secondary prevention of infarction.

417. The answer is b. *(NCEP ATP III, pp 2486–2490.)* The National Cholesterol Education Program Adult Treatment Panel III primary prevention guidelines include lowering the LDL to less than 160 if the patient is free of coronary heart disease and with zero or one risk factor. Less than 130 is recommended if free of coronary heart disease and with two or more risk factors. These risk factors include cigarette smoking, hypertension (BP 140/90 or greater, or an antihypertensive medication), low HDL cholesterol (<40 mg/dL), family history of premature coronary heart disease (CHD in first-degree male relative <55 years or in female <65 years old), age (men 45 years old or greater; women 55 or greater), and diabetes (which is regarded as a CHD equivalent requiring LDL goal <100). The goal is less than 100 in the presence of known coronary heart disease. In this example, although the patient is healthy, he has two risk factors by virtue of being male age 45 years or older, plus family history of early coronary heart disease.

418. The answer is e. *(Fuster, 10/e, pp 1142–1147.)* Of this group of choices, only exercise has been shown to raise HDL. Alcohol also increases the HDL level (HDL2 and HDL3 subfractions), thereby imparting some cardioprotective effect, but at the risk of cardiomyopathy, sudden death, hemorrhagic stroke, and other noncardiovascular problems among heavy drinkers. The cardiovascular system may benefit from aspirin via antiplatelet effects and folic acid/pyridoxine via lowering high homocysteine levels; after initial enthusiasm for vitamin E, more recent studies have not shown consistent cardiovascular benefit. None of these raise HDL. DHEA lowers HDL.

419. The answer is a. *(Braunwald, 15/e, pp 2250–2255.)* Hypertriglyceridemia, which is enhanced by poorly controlled diabetes, estrogen, and alcohol, predisposes to pancreatitis.

420. The answer is d. *(Braunwald, 15/e, p 2543.)* Although other possibilities need to be considered and possibly evaluated, the patient's age and symptoms are consistent with panic disorder. The diagnostic criteria for panic attack are a discrete period of intense fear or discomfort, in which four or more of the following symptoms develop abruptly and reach a peak within 10 min: palpitations, pounding heart, or accelerated heart rate; sweating; trembling or shaking; sensations of shortness of breath or smothering; feeling of choking; chest pain or discomfort; nausea or abdominal distress;

feeling dizzy, unsteady, lightheaded, or faint; derealization or depersonalization; fear of losing control or going crazy; fear of dying; paresthesias; chills or hot flushes.

421. The answer is c. (*Braunwald, 15/e, pp 1365–1366.*) This history and ECG suggest acute postviral pericarditis, in which the most likely confirmatory physical finding of those listed would be the pericardial friction rub. This may be transitory and may best be heard in expiration with patient upright or leaning forward.

422. The answer is c. (*Braunwald, 15/e, pp 834–838, 1227–1228.*) The bacterial pathogens listed usually cause acute diarrhea, sometimes bloody. They usually respond to fluoroquinolones, although some resistance is emerging, particularly with regard to *Campylobacter*. *Giardia* gives a more subacute to chronic picture as described in this patient. It responds to metronidazole therapy. *Cryptosporidium* is less common and occurs in immunocompromised patients.

423. The answer is b. (*Braunwald, 15/e, pp 786–787, 790.*) The usual immunizations may be given to an HIV-infected person, preferably as early in the course as possible, except for oral polio vaccine. OPV yields an unacceptably high risk of live virus proliferation and paralytic polio. Immunocompromised persons and their household contacts should receive inactivated poliovirus vaccine (IPV), not OPV.

424. The answer is e. (*Braunwald, 15/e, pp 784–785, 788.*) A Td (adult tetanus-diphtheria booster) should be given every 10 years. A flu shot should be given in this age group, but at the appropriate time in the fall. There is no recommendation to give the *Haemophilus* immunization in adults. This patient is not in one of the high-risk categories for hepatitis B (health care workers, homosexuals, injection drug users, those in institutions for the mentally retarded, and household contacts of hepatitis B carriers) and therefore has no specific indication to receive this series. The pneumococcal vaccine may be given again to higher-risk individuals at least 5 years after the original.

425. The answer is a. (*Braunwald, 15/e, pp 501–502, 584, 609–610.*) Neither the chest x-ray nor any other test has proven to be an effective screen for lung cancer (although spiral CT shows some promise). The digital rectal exam aids in screening for rectal and prostate cancer. Other options regarding colorectal cancer are flexible sigmoidoscopy every 5 years, colonscopy every 10 years, or double-contrast barium enema every 5 to 10 years. PSA levels, though somewhat controversial, play a role in prostate cancer screening. The physical exam remains important (for example, in detection of testicular and skin cancers), although definitive evidence regarding screening is sparse.

426. The answer is a. (*Braunwald, 15/e, pp 501–502, 574.*) For early detection of breast cancer, the American Cancer Society recommends breast self-examination monthly starting at age 20; breast physical examination every 3 years from ages 20 to 40, then yearly; and mammography every year beginning age 40. Other organizations advise mammography every 1 to 2 years from ages 40 to 50, then yearly.

427. The answer is a. (*Braunwald, 15/e, pp 501–502.*) Breast cancer is the most common of women's cancers. Mammography is still recommended yearly from age 50 upward (and every 1 to 2 years from ages 40 to 50, depending on the organization). Pap smears to screen for cervical cancer may be performed yearly, but after three consecutive normal exams this may be done less frequently. Endometrial tissue samples for uterine cancer become important at menopause if at high risk. There is no true screening test for ovarian cancer at present. CEA levels are not recommended as a colon cancer screen.

428. The answer is c. (*Braunwald, 15/e, pp 1253–1255.*) Many indices have been used to measure cardiac risk in the setting of noncardiac surgery, the most well known being the Goldman index. More recent guidelines from the American Heart Association and American College of Cardiology are fairly similar and emphasize the high-risk profile as recent MI (less than 30 days), unstable or advanced angina, severe valvular heart disease, significant arrhythmias (high-grade AV block, symptomatic ventricular arrhythmia, supraventricular arrhythmia with uncontrolled rate), and decompensated CHF. In this case the murmur of aortic stenosis is of concern. Moderate risk factors include stable angina, known coronary artery disease, compensated CHF, and diabetes mellitus. Low but not negligible risk factors include age greater than 75, rhythm not sinus, more than five

PVCs per minute, evidence of atherosclerosis, and abnormal ECG (such as LVH, LBBB, or ST abnormalities).

429. The answer is e. *(Braunwald, 15/e, p 2564.)* The CAGE screening tool for alcoholism consists of asking about alcohol-related trouble: cutting down, being annoyed by criticisms, guilt, and use of an eye-opener (i.e., alcohol consumption upon arising).

430. The answer is d. *(Braunwald, 15/e, p 2548.)* Depression is commonly encountered in the outpatient setting. Among the criteria for diagnosis are the presence during the same 2-week period of five or more of nine specific symptoms. Five of these are mentioned in the question; the other four are depressed mood, psychomotor agitation or retardation, feelings of worthlessness, and recurrent thoughts of death (or suicidal ideation).

431. The answer is c. *(PDR, 56/e, pp 1243–1248.)* Many medications can potentiate warfarin, including ciprofloxacin in the fluoroquinolone antibiotic group. The other choices do not. Nonsteroidal anti-inflammatory drugs may occasionally enhance warfarin's effect, so discontinuing naproxen, if anything, should lower the INR. Of interest is that one other increasingly seen potentiator of warfarin is the over-the-counter herbal product Ginkgo biloba.

432. The answer is a. *(Braunwald, 15/e, pp 2570–2571.)* The question of cocaine use must be raised in virtually all young adults with cardiovascular symptoms, despite a professed negative history. Therefore, a urine drug screen should be obtained early on. If this is negative, the patient might well need further cardiac evaluation, such as echocardiogram, ambulatory cardiac monitoring, and/or stress test.

433–435. The answers are 433-a, 434-d, 435-b. *(JNC VI, p 30.)* Alpha blockers improve urinary outflow (and also lower cholesterol slightly). ACE inhibitors are helpful in CHF, give renal protective effect in diabetics with proteinuria, and may be protective post-MI. Evidence is accumulating that angiotensin II receptor blockers provide these same benefits. Beta blockers are indicated post-MI and may help tremor as well as prevent migraines.

436–439. The answers are 436-d, 437-b, 438-b, and 439-a. (*JNC VI, pp 30, 43–44.*) Diuretics predispose to hyperuricemia and therefore gout; they can exacerbate hyperglycemia and must be used with caution in diabetics. Nonselective beta blockers are contraindicated in asthma and may adversely affect peripheral vascular disease, congestive heart failure, and diabetes. ACE inhibitors are contraindicated in the second and third trimesters of pregnancy due to the potential for fetal anomalies and death.

440. The answer is d. (*Braunwald, 15/e, pp 5–6.*) The principle of autonomy is an overriding issue in this patient, who is competent to make her own decisions about surgery. Consulting a psychiatrist would be inappropriate unless there is some reason to believe the patient is not competent. No such concern is present in this description of the patient. Since the patient is competent, no friend or relative can give permission for the procedure.

441. The answer is b. (*Braunwald, 15/e, pp 2593–2594.*) Although there is no clue to exposure (insecticides, rodenticide, wood preservatives), the clinical picture is characteristic of arsenic poisoning. Manifestations of toxicity are varied but include irritation of the GI tract, resulting in the symptoms described. Arsenic combines with the globin chain of hemoglobin to produce hemolysis. The white transverse lines of the fingernails, called Aldrich-Mees lines, are a manifestation of chronic arsenic poisoning.

442. The answer is b. (*Braunwald, 15/e, pp 2624–2625.*) Bites due to *Loxosceles* spiders (including the brown recluse) may cause necrosis of tissue at the site of the bite. The cause of the local reaction is not well understood but is thought to involve complement-mediated tissue damage. Dapsone, steroids, and antivenin have all been used in treatment, but no therapy is of proven value. The bite of the black widow spider causes neurologic signs and abdominal pain but does not result in soft tissue damage. Without fever and toxicity, the skin signs described are not likely to be secondary to bacterial infection.

443. The answer is b. (*Braunwald, 15/e, pp 5–7.*) The patient's autonomy as directed by the living will must be respected. This autonomy is not transferred to a surrogate decision maker, even one who is very credible. A family conference in this case would not change the overriding issue—that a valid living will is in effect.

444. The answer is b. (*Braunwald, 15/e, pp 2626–2627.*) The administration of epinephrine is the best treatment in the acute setting. Epinephrine provides both α- and β-adrenergic effects. Antihistamines and corticosteroids are frequently given as well, although they have little immediate effect. The patient should be offered venom immunotherapy after recovery from the systemic reaction. Removal without compression of an insect stinger is worthwhile, but not the primary concern.

445. The answer is b. (*Braunwald, 15/e, pp 2270–2271.*) Asymptomatic hyperuricemia does increase the risk of acute gouty arthritis. However, the cost of lifelong prophylaxis in this patient would be high, and the prevalence of adverse drug reaction would be between 10 and 25%. This expense is generally considered high compared to a more conservative approach of treating an attack when it does occur. Prophylactic therapy would be reserved for patients who already had one or more acute attacks. Although hyperuricemia is associated with arteriosclerotic disease, the association is not felt to be causal, and there is no proven cardiovascular benefit to reducing the uric acid level. In patients with lymphoproliferative disease, prophylaxis for the prevention of renal impairment is recommended. The risk of urolithiasis is sufficiently low that prophylaxis is not necessary until the development of a stone.

446–451. The answers are 446-a, 447-a, 448-e, 449-c, 450-b, 451-a. (*Braunwald, 15/e, pp 1031–1034.*) Recommendations for isoniazid prophylaxis include the following (based on tuberculin reaction). HIV-infected person, 5 mm or greater (duration of therapy, 12 months); close contacts of tuberculosis patients, 5 mm or greater (treat for 6 months; for child, 9 months); persons with fibrotic lesions on CXR, 5 mm or greater (treat for 12 months); recently infected persons, 10 mm or greater (treat for 6 months); Persons with high-risk medical conditions, 10 mm or greater (treat for 6 to 12 months) [includes diabetes mellitus, those on steroids or other immunosuppressive therapy, some hematologic and reticuloendothelial diseases, injectable drug use (HIV-negative), end-stage renal disease, rapid weight loss]; high-risk group (<35 years old), 10 mm or greater (treat for 6 months) (includes those from high-prevalence countries, those in medically underserved low-income populations, residents of long-term-care facilities); low-risk group (<35 years old), 15 mm or greater (treat for 6 months). By these criteria, the HIV-infected person, the 30-year-old hospital employee (low-risk or perhaps even high-risk in this example), and the 60-year-old recent converter are all candidates for isoniazid prophylaxis. The risk of developing active TB in the HIV-infected group is 5 to 10% per year and in other recent converters about 3% within the year. INH prophylaxis is most likely to be effective when infection (conversion) is recent. Consideration should be given to providing prophylaxis to all those under age 35 with positive PPDs, since the incidence of INH hepatitis in this group is low. The 40-year-old male with a positive PPD does not fall into any category of INH prophylaxis. In contrast, the new nursing home patient should get a second PPD placed in 2 weeks. About 15% of these patients will have a false-negative PPD on the first test, but a true-positive on the second. The 50-year-old Hodgkin's disease patient has active tuberculosis and must be treated with a three- or four-drug regimen. The two-drug regimen is inadequate in light of emerging resistance.

Allergy and Immunology

Questions

DIRECTIONS: Each item below contains a question or incomplete statement followed by suggested responses. Select the **one best** response to each question.

452. A 20-year-old female develops urticaria that lasts for 6 weeks and then resolves spontaneously. She gives no history of weight loss, fever, rash, or tremulousness. Physical exam shows no abnormalities. The most likely cause of the urticaria is

a. Connective tissue disease
b. Hyperthyroidism
c. Chronic infection
d. Not likely to be determined

453. A 20-year-old male is found to have weight loss and generalized lymphadenopathy. He has hypogammaglobulinemia with a normal distribution of immunoglobulin isotypes. Histologic exam of lymphoid tissue shows germinal center hyperplasia. A diagnosis of common variable immunodeficiency is made. Which of the following is correct?

a. The patient likely had symptoms in childhood
b. At least one parent is also afflicted with the disease
c. The patient may develop recurrent bronchitis and chronic idiopathic diarrhea
d. The patient should receive the standard vaccine protocol

454. A 25-year-old female complains of watery rhinorrhea and pruritus of the eyes and nose that occurs around the same season each year. Symptoms are not exacerbated by weather changes, emotion, or irritants. She is on no medications and is not pregnant. Which of the following statements is correct?

a. In this patient, symptoms are being produced by an IgE antibody against a specific allergen
b. The patient has vasomotor rhinitis
c. The patient's nasal turbinates are likely to be very red
d. Avoidance measures alone are almost always effective

455. A 20-year-old nursing student complains of asthma while on her surgical rotation. She has developed dermatitis of her hands. Symptoms are worsened when she is in the operating room. Which of the following is correct?

a. This is an allergic reaction that is always benign
b. The patient should be evaluated for latex allergy by skin testing or demonstration of specific IgE antibody
c. This syndrome is less common now than 10 years ago
d. Oral corticosteroid is indicated

Items 456–457

456. A 30-year-old male develops skin rash, pruritus, and mild wheezing about 20 min after an intravenous pyelogram performed for the evaluation of renal stone symptoms. The best approach to diagnosis of this patient includes

a. Perform 24-h urinary histamine measurement
b. Measure immunoglobulin E to radiocontrast media
c. Diagnose radiocontrast media sensitivity by history
d. Recommend intradermal skin testing

457. Appropriate acute management for this patient includes

a. Subcutaneous epinephrine for mild to moderate bronchospasm
b. Intravenous fluids
c. Prophylactic atropine
d. Diazepam to prevent seizures

DIRECTIONS: Each group of questions below consists of lettered options followed by a set of numbered items. For each numbered item, select the **one** lettered option with which it is **most** closely associated. Each lettered option may be used once, more than once, or not at all.

Items 458–460

For each clinical description, select the one most likely immunologic deficiency.

a. Wiskott-Aldrich syndrome
b. Ataxia telangiectasia
c. DiGeorge syndrome
d. Immunoglobulin A deficiency
e. Severe combined immunodeficiency
f. C1 inhibitor deficiency
g. Decay-accelerating factor deficiency

458. Recurrent episodes of nonpruritic, nonerythematous angioedema **(SELECT 1 IMMUNE DEFICIENCY)**

459. Episodes of intravascular hemolytic anemia **(SELECT 1 IMMUNE DEFICIENCY)**

460. Development of lymphoreticular neoplasm in a patient with episodes of eczema, thrombocytopenia, and recurrent infections **(SELECT 1 IMMUNE DEFICIENCY)**

461. A 40-year-old white woman with a history of chronic otitis and sinusitis is found to have a serum IgA level of 1 mg/dL. All other immunoglobulin classes are found to be normal. Which of the following statements is correct?

a. She may suffer an anaphylactic reaction following the administration of serum products
b. Clinical improvement follows regular infusions of fresh plasma
c. Infection with *Giardia* should suggest a different diagnosis
d. The disease is more common in blacks and Asians than it is in whites
e. An associated autoimmune disorder would be very rare

462. A 55-year-old farmer develops recurrent cough, dyspnea, fever, and myalgia several hours after entering his barn. Which of the following statements is true?

a. Testing of pulmonary function several hours after an exposure will most likely reveal an obstructive pattern
b. Immediate-type IgE hypersensitivity is involved in the pathogenesis of his illness
c. The etiological agents may well be thermophilic actinomycete antigens
d. Demonstrating precipitable antibodies to the offending antigen confirms the diagnosis of hypersensitivity pneumonitis

463. A 35-year-old woman is concerned that she may be allergic to some foods. She believes that she gets a rash several hours after eating small amounts of peanuts. In evaluating this concern, which of the following is correct?

a. At least 30% of the adult population is allergic to some food substance
b. Symptoms occur hours after ingestion of the food substance
c. The foods most likely to cause allergic reactions include egg, milk, seafood, nuts, and soybeans
d. The organ systems most frequently involved in allergic reactions to foods in adults are the respiratory and cardiovascular systems
e. Immunotherapy is a proven therapy for food allergies

464. A 32-year-old woman experiences a severe anaphylactic reaction following a sting from a hornet. Which of the following statements is correct?

a. She would not have a similar reaction to a sting from a yellow jacket
b. She would have a prior history of an adverse reaction to an insect sting
c. Adults are unlikely to die as a result of an insect sting compared to children with the same history
d. She should be skin-tested with venom antigens and, if positive, immunotherapy should be started

Items 465–468

For each immunologic deficiency, select the most likely infectious process that might result.

a. Complement deficiency C5–C9
b. Selective IgA deficiency
c. Post-splenectomy
d. Neutropenia
e. Interleukin 12 receptor deficit
f. Microbicidal leukocyte defect

465. Recurrent meningococcemia **(SELECT 1 IMMUNOLOGIC DEFICIENCY)**

466. *Streptococcus pneumoniae* sepsis **(SELECT 1 IMMUNOLOGIC DEFICIENCY)**

467. Disseminated apergillosis **(SELECT 1 IMMUNOLOGIC DEFICIENCY)**

468. Disseminated mycobacteria **(SELECT 1 IMMUNOLOGIC DEFICIENCY)**

Allergy and Immunology

Answers

452. The answer is d. *(Braunwald, 15/e, pp 1917–1918.)* In the great majority of patients with urticaria, a cause is never found. Some do have underlying illnesses such as chronic infection, myeloproliferative disease, collagen vascular disease, or hyperthyroidism. There is no evidence for underlying disease in this patient.

453. The answer is c. *(Stobo, 23/e, pp 677–678.)* Patients with common variable immunodeficiency syndrome usually develop recurrent or chronic infections of the respiratory or gastrointestinal tract. Patients have hypogammaglobulinemia, often with associated T cell abnormalities. Diarrhea can be idiopathic, with malabsorption, or secondary to chronic infection such as giardiasis. There is no typical genetic predisposition, although clusters in families do occur. Symptoms generally do not occur until the second or third decade of life, but also may first present in the older patient. Patients with common variable immunodeficiency syndrome should not receive live vaccines such as those for mumps, rubella, or polio.

454. The answer is a. *(Braunwald, 15/e, pp 1920–1921.)* Allergic rhinitis is caused by allergens that trigger a local hypersensitivity reaction. Specific IgE antibodies are produced and attach to circulating mast cells or basophils. Mast cell degranulation leads to a cascade of inflammatory mediators. Vasomotor rhinitis, the second most common cause of rhinitis after allergic disease, is usually perennial and is not associated with itching. In allergic rhinitis, nasal turbinates appear pale and boggy. Avoidance measures alone are often ineffective. Antihistamines and intranasal corticosteroids are usually recommended.

455. The answer is b. *(Hurst, 4/e, pp 187–189.)* Latex allergy has become an increasingly recognized problem. This is an IgE-mediated sensitivity to latex products, particularly surgical gloves. Patients present with localized urticaria at the site of contact, but can also have generalized urticaria, flushing, wheezing, laryngeal edema, and hypotension. Skin testing with latex extract confirms the diagnosis, but has caused systemic local reactions. Serum testing is definitive, but is positive in 55 to 80% of patients. Education and avoidance of latex products is the best approach to management.

456. The answer is c. *(Hurst, 4/e, pp 192–195.)* Signs and symptoms of radiocontrast media sensitivity include tachycardia, wheezing, urticaria, facial edema, bradycardia, and hypotension. When these occur within 20 min of the injection of a radiocontrast agent, the diagnosis is made by history. No routine laboratory abnormalities are diagnostic or predictive. Specific immunoglobulin E antibodies have not been identified, and no specific skin test is available.

457. The answer is a. *(Braunwald, 15/e, p 1916.)* Subcutaneous epinephrine is recommended for mild to moderate bronchospasm. (For severe bronchospasm, intravenous epinephrine might be used in this patient, who does not have contraindications.) Intravenous fluids would be recommended only when hypotension is present. Atropine is given only in the setting of bradycardia. Diazepam is used when seizures occur acutely as part of the hypersensitivity reaction.

458–460. The answers are 458-f, 459-g, 460-a. *(Braunwald, 15/e, pp 691, 1850, 1918.)* C1 inhibitor deficiency prevents the proper regulation of activated C1. As a consequence, levels of C2 and C4—substrates of C1—are also low. Recurrent angioedema is the result of uncontrolled action of other serum proteins normally controlled by C1 inhibitor. Decay-accelerating factor is a membrane-anchored protein that inhibits complement activation of host tissue. Deficiency predisposes to erythrocyte lysis that results in paroxysmal nocturnal hemoglobinuria. Wiskott-Aldrich syndrome is an X-linked recessive disorder associated with thrombocytopenia, eczema, and recurrent infection. There is an increased incidence of lymphoreticular neoplasm. The disease is the result of an abnormal protein present in platelets and the cytoplasm of peripheral mononuclear cells. Ataxia telangiectasia is an autosomal recessive immunodeficiency disorder that results in recurrent infection and malignancy but does not involve platelet abnormalities. It is also the result of an abnormally encoded protein.

461. The answer is a. (*Braunwald, 15/e, p 1848.*) IgA deficiency occurs in approximately 1 of 700 births. It is much more common in whites than in blacks or Asians. (The incidence in Japan is 1 in 18,500.) IgA-deficient patients produce autoantibodies. Some develop high levels of antibody to IgA, which can result in anaphylactic reaction when transfused with normal blood or blood products. Failure to produce IgA antibody results in recurrent upper respiratory tract infections in more than 50% of affected patients. Chronic diarrhea and *Giardia* infection are common problems. IgA-deficient patients frequently have autoimmune disorders, atopic problems, and malabsorption and eventually develop pulmonary disease. IgA cannot be effectively replaced with exogenous immunoglobulin.

462. The answer is c. (*Braunwald, 15/e, pp 1463–1465.*) Hypersensitivity pneumonitis is characterized by an immunologic inflammatory reaction in response to inhaling organic dusts, the most common of which are thermophilic actinomycetes, fungi, and avian proteins. In the acute form of the illness, exposure to the offending antigen is intense. Cough, dyspnea, fever, chills, and myalgia, which typically occur 4 to 8 hours after exposure, are the presenting symptoms. In the subacute form, antigen exposure is moderate, chills and fever are usually absent, and cough, anorexia, weight loss, and dyspnea dominate the presentation. In the chronic form of hypersensitivity pneumonitis, progressive dyspnea, weight loss, and anorexia are seen; pulmonary fibrosis is a noted complication. The finding of IgG antibody to the offending antigen is universal, although it may be present in asymptomatic patients as well and is therefore not diagnostic. While peripheral T cell, B cell, and monocyte counts are normal, a suppressor cell functional defect can be demonstrated in these patients. Inhalation challenge with the suspected antigen and concomitant testing of pulmonary function help to confirm the diagnosis. Therapy involves avoidance; steroids are administered in severe cases. Bronchodilators and antihistamines are not effective.

463. The answer is c. (*Hurst, 4/e, pp 183–185.*) Food allergy is an IgE-mediated reaction to antigens in food. It is caused by glycoproteins found in shellfish, peanuts, eggs, milk, nuts, and soybeans. Symptoms occur within minutes of ingestion in most patients. The incidence of true food allergy in the general population is uncertain but is likely to be about 1% of patients—less than might be generally perceived. Studies have demonstrated that exclusive breastfeeding can decrease the incidence of allergies to food in infants genetically predisposed to developing them. Food allergens cause symptoms most commonly expressed in the gastrointestinal tract and the skin. In addition, respiratory and (in severe reactions) cardiovascular symptoms may occur. Food allergic reactions are diagnosed by the medical history, skin tests, or radioallergosorbent tests (RASTs), and elimination diets. The best test, however, remains the double-blind, placebo-controlled food challenge. If the diagnosis of a food allergy is confirmed, the only proven therapy is avoidance of the offending food. At present, there is no role for immunotherapy in the treatment of food allergy.

464. The answer is d. (*Braunwald, 15/e, pp 2626–2627.*) The incidence of insect sting allergy is difficult to determine. Approximately 40 deaths per year occur as a result of *Hymenoptera* stings. Additional fatalities undoubtedly occur and are unknowingly attributed to other causes. Both atopic and nonatopic persons experience reactions to insect stings. The responses range from large local reactions with erythema and swelling at the sting site to acute anaphylaxis. The majority of fatal reactions occur in adults, with most persons having had no previous reaction to a stinging insect. Reactions can occur with the first sting and usually begin within 15 min. Enzymes, biogenic amines, and peptides are the allergens present in the insects' venom that provoke allergic reactions. Venoms are commercially available for testing and treatment. Within the *Vespidae* family, which consists of hornets, yellow jackets, and wasps, cross-sensitivity to the various insect venoms occurs. The honeybee, which belongs to the *Apis* family, does not show cross-reactivity with the vespids. Venom immunotherapy is indicated for patients with a history of sting anaphylaxis and positive skin tests.

465–468. The answers are 465-a, 466-c, 467-d, 468-e. (*Braunwald, 15/e, pp 366, 552, 883, 933, 1813.*) Patients who have a deficiency of one of the terminal components of complement have a remarkable susceptibility to disseminated *Neisseria* infection, particularly meningococcal disease. This association with meningococcal disease is related to the host inability to assemble what is called a membrane attack complex—a single molecule of complement components that creates a discontinuity in the bacteria's membrane lipid bilayer. The complement deficiency results in inability to express complement-dependent bactericidal activity.

The pneumococcus is the most important organism in sepsis that occurs post-splenectomy, making up about 67% of all cases. (*Haemophilus influenzae* is the second most common organism.) The spleen has a variety of immunologic functions, but, as the main production site for opsonizing antibody, it is especially important for the clearance of encapsulated bacteria. A polysaccharide capsule surrounds all invasive pneumococci, and a deficiency in opsonizing antibody post-splenectomy can result in overwhelming sepsis with pneumonia, bacteremia, meningitis, and death.

Severe neutropenia can result from hematologic malignancy, aplastic anemia, or cytotoxic chemotherapy. The risk of infection increases with the extent and duration of neutropenia. Below 500 cells per μL, the risk of infection rises dramatically. Early in the course of neutropenia, bacteremia from gram-negative bacteria such as *Pseudomonas aeruginosa* is common. In patients who have received antibiotics, fungemia is the major risk, particularly from *Aspergillus* or *Candida* species. Disseminated *Aspergillus* almost always occurs in the setting of severe neutropenia. Disseminated mycobacterial infection has recently been linked to patients who have interleukin 12 receptor deficiency. IL-12 is a monocyte-macrophage product that acts on lymphocytes to produce interferon γ. The diagnosis is made by molecular assay, and patients have been treated with interferon γ.

Geriatrics

Questions

DIRECTIONS: Each item below contains a question or incomplete statement followed by suggested responses. Select the **one best** response to each question.

469. An 80-year-old male with mild Alzheimer's disease has been started on donepezil 5 mg after he continued to have difficulty in financial matters and keeping track of the day of the week and time. After 3 months the family feels that there has been no improvement. There are no complaints of nausea, dizziness, or hypotension. The patient's wife feels the medication is unnecessary. The best advice is

a. Discontinue donepezil
b. Increase the donepezil dose to 10 mg
c. Continue donepezil to prevent further plaque formation
d. Continue donepezil for 3 to 6 months and reevaluate mental status
e. Begin a new anticholinesterase inhibitor

470. A 78-year-old woman with mild renal insufficiency complains of pain in the right knee on walking that has interfered with her day-to-day activities. Pain is relieved by rest. There are no inflammatory symptoms of redness or swelling. There is minimal joint effusion. An x-ray of the knee shows osteophytes and asymmetric loss of joint space. ESR and white blood cell count are normal. The best initial management of this patient is

a. Nonsteroidal anti-inflammatory agent
b. Intraarticular corticosteroids
c. Acetaminophen
d. Total arthroplasty

471. An 82-year-old man complains of 2 h of severe chest pain that occurred while he was playing tennis. Blood pressure on admission is 140/70, and heart rate is 110. There are no signs of congestive heart failure. Pulses are all palpable, and abdominal exam is normal. Neurologic exam is normal, and stool is guaiac-negative. There is no history of gastrointestinal bleeding, previous stroke, head trauma, or major surgery. There is no history of vascular disease or liver disease. ECG shows ST segment elevation of 3 mm in leads V1–V3, with three premature ventricular beats per minute. The initial treatment of choice is

a. Prophylactic lidocaine
b. Thrombolytic therapy and aspirin
c. Heparin
d. Aspirin alone

472. A 65-year-old man has had symptoms of progressive cognitive dysfunction over a 1-year period. Memory and calculation ability are worsening. The patient has also had episodes of paranoia and delusions. Antipsychotic medication resulted in extrapyramidal signs and was stopped. The patient has recently complained of several months of visual hallucinations. There is no history of alcohol abuse. The most likely diagnosis is

a. Lewy body dementia
b. Alzheimer's disease
c. Early parkinsonism
d. Delirium

473. An 80-year-old nursing home patient has become increasingly confused and unstable on her feet. On one occasion she has wandered outside the nursing home. In considering the issue of restraints for this individual, which of the following is correct?

a. A geri-chair would provide the best approach to safety and restraint
b. Physical restraints are the best methods to prevent falls
c. Restraints cause many complications and increase the risk of falls
d. Sedative medication should be used instead of restraints

474. A 75-year-old woman who is living independently seeks advice about exercise programs. She has mild hypertension but is otherwise in good health with no other risk factors for cardiovascular disease. Which of the following statements is supported by current data?

a. Walking can reduce mortality from cardiovascular disease and help prevent falls
b. Tai chi has become popular in the elderly but results in falls
c. This patient would require stress testing before beginning a walking program
d. Only high-intensity exercise has been shown to have long-standing benefits

475. A frail 80-year-old nursing home resident has had several episodes of syncope, all of which have occurred while she was returning to her room after breakfast. She complains of light-headedness and states she feels cold and weak. She takes nitroglycerin in the morning for a history of chest pain, but denies recent chest pain or shortness of breath. The most likely method of diagnosis is

a. Cardiac catheterization
b. Postprandial blood pressure monitoring
c. Holter monitoring
d. CT scan

476. A 70-year-old woman complains of insomnia and feeling sad. Her husband died 2 months ago, and she has had these symptoms since the funeral. She feels guilty that she did not care for her husband well enough. She has recently moved to a smaller apartment. She denies weight loss or functional impairment. On occasion, she has thought she heard her husband's voice. The best approach to management is

a. Hospitalization and suicide precautions
b. Antipsychotic medication
c. Bereavement support for at least 1 year
d. Treatment for major depression

477. Which of the following medications should be avoided in the elderly for the indication given?

a. A beta blocker after myocardial infarction
b. Angiotensin converting enzyme inhibitor in left ventricular systolic dysfunction
c. Warfarin in chronic atrial fibrillation
d. Digoxin in early signs of congestive heart failure

478. A 78-year-old male complains of slowly progressive hearing loss. He finds it particularly difficult to hear his grandchildren and to appreciate conversation in a crowded restaurant. On exam, ear canal and tympanic membranes are normal. Audiology testing finds bilateral upper-frequency hearing loss with difficulties in speech discrimination. The most likely diagnosis is

a. Presbycusis
b. Cerumen impaction
c. Ménière's disease
d. Chronic otitis media

479. Many physiologic changes are associated with aging. Which of the following physiologic parameters does not change with age?

a. Creatinine clearance
b. Forced expiratory volume
c. Hematocrit
d. Heart rate response to stress
e. Hours of REM sleep

480. A 65-year-old male who has not had routine medical care presents for a physical exam and is found to have a blood pressure of 165/80. He has no other risk factors for heart disease. He is not obese and walks 1 mile a day. Physical exam shows no retinopathy, normal cardiac exam including point of maximal impulse, and normal pulses. There is no abdominal bruit, and neurological exam is normal. ECG, electrolytes, blood sugar, and urinalysis are also normal. Repeat visit 2 weeks later shows blood pressure to be unchanged. The next step in management is

a. Do a workup for secondary causes, including intravenous pyelogram
b. Begin therapy with a low-dose diuretic
c. Follow patient; avoid toxicity of antihypertensive agents
d. Begin therapy with a beta blocker

481. A 65-year-old male inquires about the pneumonia vaccine. He has a friend who died of pneumonia. The patient is in good health without underlying disease. You should

a. Recommend the pneumococcal vaccine and check on the status of other immunizations, particularly tetanus vaccination
b. Inform the patient that he has no risk factors for pneumonia
c. Report that the present pneumonia vaccine does not work
d. Emphasize that the influenza vaccine is more important

Geriatrics

Answers

469. The answer is d. (*Hazzard, 4/e, pp 1266–1267.*) The best course would be to continue the donepezil and see if it slows progression of cognitive function loss based on mini–mental status exam or family assessment. The success of the intervention needs to be evaluated over a longer time period, realizing that success may mean maintaining baseline function. The anticholinesterase inhibitors do not prevent plaque formation. Increasing dose is rarely helpful and often causes side effects. There is no data to suggest that one anticholinesterase inhibitor works better than another.

470. The answer is c. (*Hazzard, 4/e, pp 1156–1159.*) In addition to physical therapy, the best symptomatic treatment would be acetaminophen because it is frequently effective in providing pain relief and has an excellent safety profile in the elderly. Nonsteroidals should be avoided, at least initially, because they tend to cause gastrointestinal upset and impairment of renal function. Intraarticular steroids are indicated for large effusions in joints unresponsive to first-line therapy. Arthroplasty is highly effective in treating osteoarthritis of a single joint and is not contraindicated in the elderly. Such surgery is usually considered after attempts at physical therapy, education, and pain relief with pharmacotherapy.

471. The answer is b. (*Hazzard, 4/e, p 944.*) The patient has clinical and ECG evidence for acute myocardial infarction. He has no contraindications to thrombolytic therapy. (Age per se is not a contraindication to thrombolytic therapy.) Thirty-day mortality is markedly decreased for elderly patients with acute MI treated with aspirin and thrombolytic therapy. Many elderly patients, of course, will have contraindications to thrombolytics, particularly gastrointestinal bleeding, recent stroke, head injury, or surgery. Aspirin alone is not as effective in reducing mortality. Antiarrthymic agents do not reduce mortality and have pronounced side effects in the elderly. Heparin should be given following thrombolytic therapy.

472. The answer is a. (*Braunwald, 15/e, pp 151, 2396.*) Lewy body dementia has been recently recognized as a specific type of dementia different from

Alzheimer's disease or Parkinson's disease. On autopsy there is evidence of Lewy bodies throughout the brain, including the cortex. Mild parkinsonism may or may not be present. Paranoia and delusions are more common than in Alzheimer's disease, and treatment with antipsychotic drugs characteristically worsens the underlying condition. The visual hallucinations are the most characteristic clinical symptom, making the diagnosis of Alzheimer's disease less likely. Delirium is an acute confusional state that would not present with progressive cognitive deterioration or repeated hallucinations over time.

473. The answer is c. *(Kane, 4/e, pp 252–253.)* Restraints are being used less and less in nursing homes as their complications and alternatives become more appreciated. The **four D's**—**d**econditioning, **d**epression, **d**isorientation, and **d**ecubiti—are all complications of restraints. A geri-chair is just another form of physical restraint, which promotes the same difficulties. Effective alternatives to restraints usually require an individual care plan. In this case, alarm bells for the institution's exits and evaluation of the patient's gait would be important. Sedation leads to complications such as pneumonia and may, in fact, also promote falls.

474. The answer is a. *(Hazzard, 4/e, pp 295–298.)* Walking is the most common exercise in the elderly and has been shown to reduce mortality from coronary artery disease and decrease the incidence of falls. In one study, a rigorous walking program of 2 miles a day reduced coronary artery disease events by 50%. Tai chi exercises, which consist of a sequence of movements used in martial arts, have actually been shown to reduce the incidence of falls in older patients. Exercise need not be high-intensity to have benefits; moderate-intensity activity for 30 min produces most of the health benefits of daily exercise. Judgment dictates the degree of medical screening and the use of exercise stress testing in elderly patients who are beginning an exercise program. A walking program does not require such screening. Exercise stress testing has been recommended by some experts for elderly patients with two or more risk factors for heart disease.

475. The answer is b. *(Hazzard, 4/e, pp 1529–1532.)* Postprandial hypotension has been increasingly recognized in the frail elderly. Postprandial reduction in systolic blood pressure in the elderly is common. In one study, a quarter of all patients had a reduction in systolic blood pressure of greater than 20 mmHg. Much of the decrease is due to splanchnic blood pooling. Those on nitrates and other drugs that cause postural hypotension are at greatest risk. Older patients with this condition should avoid large meals. Diagnosis is confirmed by monitoring blood pressure after eating. Cardiac ischemia or arrythmia cannot be ruled out but are less likely to cause the symptoms described. Arrythmia is more likely to be of sudden onset but could be evaluated by continuous monitoring later in the workup. CT scan is rarely helpful in the evaluation of syncope in a patient without focal neurologic findings.

476. The answer is c. *(Kane, 4/e, p 169.)* This patient presents with typical characteristics of a bereavement reaction. Symptoms of guilt, insomnia, and loss are occurring within 1 year of the spouse's death. There are no symptoms of a major depression. It is not uncommon to have transient hallucinations of hearing the spouse's voice; this does not represent psychosis and does not require medication. Antidepressants can usually be avoided, and indeed may interfere with the process of adjustment. Counseling and supportive services such as widows' groups facilitate the transition period. The physician should be aware of any clues to decline in health, common during this period. The patient should be followed for suicidal ideation.

477. The answer is d. *(Kane, 4/e, p 314.)* All medications should be carefully considered in the elderly with respect to side effects and drug interactions. However, some medications are in fact used too infrequently in the elderly because of side effect concerns. Beta blockers prolong survival in the elderly after myocardial infarction, and have probably been used too infrequently in the elderly after MI. Similarly, ACE inhibitors have a beneficial effect on mortality and functional status in the elderly with systolic function. They should be prescribed unless there are contraindications such as intolerance, renal insufficiency, elevated serum potassium, or hypotension. Warfarin reduces the risk of thromboembolic events in the elderly with atrial fibrillation. It is estimated that warfarin could prevent an additional 40,000 strokes per year in patients with atrial fibrillation, most of whom are elderly. Digoxin is rarely a drug of choice for heart failure in the elderly patient. In general, it is a drug to avoid in the elderly because of its toxic-to-therapeutic ratio and tendency for drug interactions.

478. The answer is a. (*Hazzard, 4/e, pp 617–628.*) Presbycusis is the most common cause of sensorineural hearing loss in the elderly. Probably the result of cochlear damage over time, it is characterized by bilateral high-frequency hearing loss above 2000 Hz. Diminished speech discrimination is more apparent as compared to other causes of hearing loss. Both Ménière's disease and chronic otitis media are common causes of hearing loss in the elderly; they usually present as unilateral hearing loss. Otoscopy should always be used to rule out hearing loss due to cerumen impaction in the elderly patient.

479. The answer is c. (*Braunwald, 15/e, p 38.*) Hematocrit does not vary with age, and elderly patients with anemia require workup to define the disease process. Lung elasticity decreases with age, resulting in some change over time in pulmonary function test. Creatinine clearance decreases with age, as do heart rate response to stress and number of hours of REM sleep.

480. The answer is b. (*Kane, 4/e, pp 296–297.*) There is now general agreement that systolic hypertension in the elderly should be treated and that low-dose thiazide diuretic is the initial regimen of choice in the elderly. Treatment reduces the risk of stroke and cardiovascular events, and side effects appear to be minimal. Low-dose reserpine or atenolol are generally recommended as second-step therapy. Workup for secondary causes is not indicated as they are less common in the elderly; however, such a workup may be appropriate if hypertension is refractory to medication. Weight loss and exercise might be initiated prior to antihypertensive medication in a patient with mild systolic hypertension who is obese or sedentary.

481. The answer is a. (*Braunwald, 15/e, p 45.*) The pneumococcal vaccine is currently recommended for all patients over the age of 65 because age per se is a risk factor for mortality due to pneumococcal infection. The vaccine is safe, and the vaccination program for the elderly is cost-effective. The importance of the annual influenza vaccine should also be explained to the patient. If the visit is during influenza season, both vaccines should be given at the same time. Tetanus vaccination booster is also recommended in the elderly patient who has not had a booster vaccine in 10 years.

Women's Health

Questions

DIRECTIONS: Each item below contains a question or incomplete statement followed by suggested responses. Select the **one best** response to each question.

Items 482–484

A 20-year-old sexually active female presents for an annual exam. She tells you she has had four sexual partners in the past, she has participated in unprotected intercourse sometimes, and her age at first coitus was 15. She has a 5-pack-year tobacco history. Her family history is positive for early coronary artery disease in her father and paternal grandfather. On physical exam, she is overweight. Otherwise her exam is normal. On pelvic exam, there are no cervical lesions, and a Pap smear is obtained.

482. Which of the following screening tests is recommended for this patient?

a. Liver function tests
b. Chest x-ray
c. Mammogram
d. Lipid profile

483. Several days later, the Pap smear result is reported as a low-grade squamous intraepithelial lesion (LGSIL). Which infectious agent is most likely associated with this result?

a. Human papillomavirus (HPV)
b. Herpes simplex virus
c. Chlamydia
d. *Trichomonas vaginalis*

484. Based on the above information, this patient should

a. Have further evaluation of cervical abnormality
b. Have an annual Pap smear
c. Have a repeat Pap smear if and when she changes sexual partners
d. Have Pap smear repeated every 3 years

Items 485–487

A 60-year-old white female presents for an office visit. Her mother recently broke her hip, and the patient is concerned about her own risk for osteoporosis. She weighs 165 lb and is 5 ft, 6 in. tall. She has a 50-pack-year history of tobacco use. Medications include a multivitamin and levothyroxine 50 μg/d. Her exercise regimen includes mowing the lawn and taking care of the garden. She took hormone replacement therapy for 6 years after menopause, which occurred at age 49.

485. Which test related to osteoporosis, if any, is appropriate for this patient?

a. Nuclear medicine bone scan
b. Dual x-ray absorptiometry (Dexa scan)
c. No testing is required at this time
d. Peripheral bone densitometry

486. In counseling this patient about osteoporosis, you should advise her that she might benefit from

a. Fluoride supplementation
b. Calcium supplementation
c. Continuing her current exercise routine
d. Restarting hormone replacement therapy

487. Which of the following contributes to the development of osteoporosis?

a. Family history of osteoporosis
b. Hypothyroidism
c. Obesity
d. Use of hormone replacement therapy

Items 488–489

A 50-year-old woman presents with a vague complaint of fatigue and dyspnea on exertion. The dyspnea occurs with activities such as vacuuming or climbing the stairs in her home. Resting for 10 to 15 min relieves the symptoms. The patient noticed this about 1 to 2 months ago. She denies chest pain, orthopnea, paroxysmal nocturnal dyspnea, or recent respiratory infection. Past medical history is significant for hypertension for 10 years and hyperlipidemia for 5 years. Her medications include hydrochlorothiazide. She tries to watch her cholesterol intake. Social history is negative for tobacco use. She does recall a family history of heart attacks and strokes in her mother's family, but cannot give details. On physical exam, lungs are clear bilaterally and cardiovascular exam is unremarkable without murmurs. A left carotid bruit is noted. ECG reveals poor R wave progression in V1–V2 and nonspecific ST-T wave changes anterolaterally. Chest x-ray is normal. Pulse oximetry is 97%. Laboratory evaluation shows a normal complete blood count, cholesterol 250, HDL 29 mg/dL, LDL 160 mg/dL, glucose (random) 250/dL.

488. Which of the following disease processes might be contributing to this patient's symptoms?

a. Coronary artery disease
b. Pneumonia
c. Medication side effects
d. Anxiety disorder

489. Which of the following actions would be most helpful in the diagnosis of this patient?

a. Discontinuation of current medication
b. Pulmonary function testing
c. Graded exercise treadmill stress test
d. Graded exercise treadmill stress test with thallium scanning
e. No further test necessary, reassure the patient

Items 490–491

A 55-year-old white female presents for an annual exam. Medical history is significant for hypertension. She is a nonsmoker. Family history is negative for coronary artery disease. She has no acute complaints. She weighs 80 kg and is 1.65 m tall. BP is 150/100, cholesterol 250 mg/dL, triglycerides 300 mg/dL, HDL 30 mg/dL, and LDL 160 mg/dL.

490. This patient's calculated body mass index (BMI) is

a. 33
b. 29
c. 25
d. 22.4
e. 20

491. An acceptable BMI is

a. <21
b. <22
c. <23
d. <24
e. <25

Items 492–494

A 28-year-old female complains of fatigue and a sense of fullness at the base of her neck. She has no significant past medical history, gave birth to a healthy infant 4 months ago, and is only taking oral contraceptives. On exam, vital signs are pulse 88, blood pressure 110/66, temperature 98.6° F, and respirations 12. You note a homogeneously enlarged thyroid gland and a very mild fine tremor. The rest of the exam is within normal limits. Laboratory evaluation reveals the following:

WBC: 7.8
Hgb: 12.3
Hct: 36
Plt: 220
Na: 138
K: 4.0
Cl: 106
CO_2: 26
BUN: 12
Creatinine: 0.7
TSH: 0.01
T_4: 19
Antithyroid antibody test: elevated

492. Preliminary diagnosis is consistent with

a. Thyrotoxicosis factitia
b. Subacute thyroiditis
c. Toxic multinodular goiter
d. Postpartum thyroiditis
e. Struma ovarii

493. A thyroid uptake scan is ordered. You expect

a. Increased uptake in the thyroid gland
b. Decreased uptake in the thyroid gland
c. Multiple hot nodules
d. Not enough information to determine

494. The most appropriate next step is

a. Radioactive iodine
b. Surgical referral
c. Have the patient's family search her home for exogenous source of thyroid hormone
d. Levothyroxine 50 μg
e. Watchful waiting

Items 495–497

495. A 21-year-old female presents with complaints of dysuria for the past 48 h. She denies elevated temperature, chills, or nausea/vomiting. She states she is having some difficulty sleeping at night. She is 28 weeks pregnant with her first child. You note she is wearing long sleeves in warm weather and she has bruising on her forearms and left lateral thoracic area. An appropriate way to explore your concerns with the patient would be to ask which of the following questions?

a. "Do you know how you got these bruises?"
b. "Who hit you?"
c. "How long has your partner been abusing you?"
d. "I will have to report these injuries to the appropriate authorities if you can't explain them."

496. A dipstick urinalysis in your office reveals 2+ leukocyte esterase, trace blood, no protein, no glucose, and 2+ nitrites. You send the urine to the laboratory for culture and sensitivity but want to start empiric treatment for the patient's symptoms. Which medication is the most appropriate?

a. Ciprofloxacin
b. Cephalexin
c. Trimethoprim-sulfamethoxazole
d. Tetracycline
e. Gentamicin

497. One month after delivery, this patient is referred back to you by her obstetrician due to the onset of fatigue, dyspnea, and lower extremity edema. By history, physical examination, and testing including cardiac echocardiogram and chest x-ray, you make the diagnosis of peripartum cardiomyopathy. Which of the following is correct?

a. Peripartum cardiomyopathy may occur unexpectedly years after pregnancy and delivery
b. The postpartum state will require a different therapeutic approach than typical treatment for dilated cardiomyopathy
c. Since the condition is idiosyncratic, future pregnancy may be entered into with no greater than average risk
d. Fifty percent of patients will completely recover

498. A 78-year-old female presents to your office for follow-up. She has a history of paroxysmal atrial fibrillation and takes warfarin and digoxin for this problem. Her complaints today are a recent 5-lb weight loss, daily fatigue, and loss of interest in her usual activities. She states she doesn't feel like getting up in the morning. Her spouse adds that she has started taking some alternative therapies from the health food store in an attempt to boost her energy level. On exam, the patient is less animated than usual, and her pulse is irregular at 120/min. She has clear lungs and 1+ edema of the lower extremities. You examine the bag of pills the spouse has brought from the medicine cabinet at home. Which medication is most likely contributing to patient's problem with rapid heart rate?

a. Ginkgo biloba
b. Multivitamin with minerals
c. St. John's wort
d. Soy estrogen
e. Ginseng

499. A 40-year-old female presents to your office regarding a breast lump she found on self-exam 2 weeks ago. The patient does not regularly examine her breasts. Her last clinical breast exam was 2 years ago, and mammogram 9 months ago was normal with recommendation for follow-up mammogram in 1 year. She has no family members with breast cancer. Her father had colon cancer diagnosed 10 years ago. She takes no medications regularly. On examination, she has a well-localized nontender nodule with irregular borders of approximately 1.5 cm in the left breast at 2:00. Repeat diagnostic breast imaging reveals a negative mammogram and solid area at 2:00 in the left breast by ultrasound. You should

a. Reassure your patient and follow up in 6 months
b. Refer the patient for surgical biopsy
c. Tell the patient to discontinue caffeine and wear a supportive bra
d. Schedule a CT scan of the thorax
e. Start the patient on NSAIDs and vitamin E

500. A 57-year-old white female with a significant past medical history of breast cancer stage 2, ER+, PR+, presents to the emergency room complaining of the sudden onset of chest pain and shortness of breath 2 h ago. The pain is sharp and stabbing in the left posterior lung area. The pain does not increase on exertion but increases with deep breathing. The patient denies any history of cardiovascular or pulmonary disease. Her only medication is tamoxifen for 2 years and OTC vitamins. Pulse is 110, RR 26, BP 150/94; lungs are clear bilaterally; cardiovascular exam shows regular rate and rhythm with a fixed split on S_2. ECG shows S wave in lead 1, Q wave in lead 3, and inverted T in lead 3.

Pulse oximetry is 90% on room air. Chest x-ray is unremarkable. What is most likely to have contributed to this patient's current respiratory distress?

a. Myocardial infarction
b. Breast cancer metastasis
c. Tamoxifen use
d. Anxiety attack
e. Pneumonia

Women's Health

Answers

482. The answer is d. (*Braunwald, 15/e, pp 21–25, 501.*) A lipid profile is recommended every 5 years for patients 20 years of age or older. With this patient's family history of early coronary artery disease, which suggests a possible dyslipidemia, a lipid profile is warranted. There is no indication in the history that screening liver function tests are required. A chest x-ray is not indicated for screening even if the patient is a tobacco user. Screening mammography is recommended for the majority of patients beginning at age 40 to 50 years, depending on specific group guidelines.

483. The answer is a. (*Braunwald, 15/e, pp 1118–1134.*) Human papillomavirus (especially subtypes 16, 18, and 31) has an established relationship to abnormal Pap smears and cervical dysplasia. HIV, *Chlamydia*, or herpesvirus infections are not directly associated with cervical dysplasia.

484. The answer is a. (*Braunwald, 15/e, p 48.*) The current recommendation for workup of abnormal cervical cytology includes repeat Pap smear at 3 to 4 months, HPV DNA typing, or colposcopy, depending on the patient and her history. A Pap smear every 3 years is acceptable for low-risk patients with three negative annual consecutive Pap smears. There is no recommendation for early repeat Pap smear if a patient has a new sexual partner. Sexually active women should have annual cervical screening, with the exception of low-risk patients, who can discuss changing the screening interval with their physician.

485. The answer is b. (*Braunwald, 15/e, pp 2230–2236.*) The World Health Organization and the National Osteoporosis Foundation agree that all postmenopausal patients who are estrogen-deficient should have a central bone densitometry. A nuclear medicine scan has no role in the diagnosis of osteoporosis. Certainly this patient with estrogen deficiency, low calcium intake, family history, and previous tobacco use has a high pretest probability of osteoporosis; therefore a peripheral bone densitometry, which is used for screening only, would not be a diagnostic test of choice. In addition, due to the above explanation, testing is justified.

486. The answer is b. *(Braunwald, 15/e, pp 2194, 2232–2234.)* Postmenopausal women not on estrogen replacement should achieve a daily intake of calcium at 1200 mg of elemental calcium. The average woman in the United States receives 600 to 700 mg from diet alone. The current recommendation is that women consume 1200 mg oral calcium supplement in two or three divided doses. Although fluoride is an osteoclast inhibitor, early studies revealed an increased fracture rate with fluoride supplementation for prevention or treatment of osteoporosis. Fluoride does not have a proven role in the prevention or treatment of osteoporosis. The current exercise regimen recommended is weight-bearing activities such as walking, dancing, tennis, or jogging three to five times per week. This patient is not performing adequate weight-bearing exercise. There is no indication at this time that the patient should restart hormone replacement therapy without further diagnostic testing. If this patient is diagnosed with osteoporosis, treatment options such as the bisphosphonates, calcitonin, selective estrogen modulators (SERMs), or hormone replacement therapy are available.

487. The answer is a. *(Braunwald, 15/e, pp 2228–2229.)* A positive family history of osteoporosis is a risk factor for the development of osteoporosis. There is a definite relationship between prolonged hyperthyroidism or over-supplementation of hypothyroid patients, but hypothyroidism per se is not associated with the development of osteoporosis. A body weight under 70 kg, not obesity, is associated with osteoporosis. Hormone replacement therapy has an FDA indication for prevention and treatment of osteoporosis and therefore is not a contributor to the development of this disease.

488. The answer is a. *(Braunwald, 15/e, pp 61, 2111, 2255, 2544.)* This patient has exercise-induced symptoms. Women may present with atypical symptoms relating to coronary artery disease. This patient has hyperlipidemia that is untreated and may have type 2 diabetes mellitus with a random glucose >200 mg/dL. These risk factors coupled with her symptoms make coronary artery disease the most likely choice. This patient's history and physical are negative for signs and symptoms relating to pneumonia. Diuretics do not contribute to dyspnea. The history is not suggestive of anxiety or panic disorder.

489. The answer is d. (*Braunwald, 15/e, p 1402.*) The most appropriate test would be a treadmill stress test with thallium imaging. A treadmill stress test has a lower sensitivity and specificity in patients with atypical or no chest pain. The overall sensitivity of exercise stress electrocardiography is about 75%. Therefore a negative treadmill stress test would not rule out coronary disease. Subsequent thallium imaging improves sensitivity and specificity.

490. The answer is b. (*Braunwald, 15/e, p 479.*) Calculated BMI-weight (kg)/height (m)^2.

491. The answer is e. (*Braunwald, 15/e, p 479.*) Data from the Metropolitan Life Tables indicate that BMIs for the midpoint of all heights and frames among both men and women range from 19 to 26 kg/m^2. Even at similar BMIs, women have more body fat than men. A BMI of 30 is most commonly used as a threshold for obesity in both men and women. This cutoff of 30 is based on unequivocal data. When BMIs are >25, the risk of all-cause, metabolic, and cardiovascular mortality rises, suggesting that the cutoff for obesity should be lowered. Some authorities use the term overweight (rather than obese) to describe individuals with BMIs between 25 or 27 and 30. A BMI between 25 and 30 should be viewed as medically significant and worthy of therapeutic intervention, especially in the presence of risk factors that are influenced by adiposity, such as hypertension and glucose intolerance. The desired BMI range is 18.5 to 24.9.

492. The answer is d. (*Braverman, 8/e, pp 578–589.*) The patient's clinical presentation is most consistent with postpartum thyroiditis, a form of autoimmune-induced thyrotoxicosis that occurs 3 to 6 months after delivery. The hyperthyroid state usually lasts for 1 to 3 months and is generally followed by a hypothyroid state of limited duration. The patient's thyroid gland would not be enlarged if she were taking exogenous thyroid medications. Subacute thyroiditis almost always presents with a tender, enlarged thyroid gland. The patient's thyroid gland is described as homogeneous, not nodular, which would be inconsistent with toxic multinodular goiter. Struma ovarii is unlikely because of the enlargement of the thyroid gland. Struma ovarii is the name given to the approximately 3% of ovarian dermoid tumors or teratomas that contain thyroid tissue. This tissue may autonomously secrete thyroid hormone.

Graves' disease is another possibility. These two abnormal thyroid states could be distinguished with thyroid uptake scan.

493. The answer is b. *(Braverman, 8/e, pp 578–589.)* Postpartum thyroiditis is an autoimmune destruction of the thyroid gland that causes release of already formed hormone. Therefore, uptake in the damaged gland is low. The thyroid scan for thyroiditis shows low RAI uptake versus Graves' disease, where the uptake is increased. In Graves' disease, autoantibodies bind to the TSH receptor and stimulate the gland to increase function and hormone output. Therefore in Graves' disease there is increased uptake on the thyroid scan.

494. The answer is e. *(Braverman, 8/e, pp 578–589.)* As 90% of cases of postpartum thyroiditis spontaneously recover after 3 to 6 months, watchful waiting is the best approach to this abnormality. Symptom management with beta blockers is reasonable, but the patient described has no tachycardia and no symptoms amenable to treatment with beta blockers at this time.

495. The answer is a. *(Carr, 1/e, pp 722–728.)* It is important to recognize the increased risk of domestic abuse during pregnancy. However, jumping to the conclusion that the patient's spouse caused her apparent injuries is not warranted. Often, a patient simply needs the opportunity to express her concerns if she is in an abusive situation.

496. The answer is b. *(Carr, 1/e, p 408.)* Empiric treatment of simple UTI in pregnancy should consider the following: coverage of probable organisms (usually *Escherichia coli*), possibility of complicating factors such as pyelonephritis or nephrolithiasis, stage of pregnancy, and relative contraindication to the antibiotic. The antibiotics listed all would cover suspected organisms in simple UTI of pregnancy. However, all but one of the antibiotics is contraindicated in pregnancy. Ciprofloxacin is pregnancy category D because of concern about cartilage formation in animal studies. Trimethoprim-sulfa is not the best choice in later stages of pregnancy because trimethoprim is a folate antagonist and is teratogenic in rats and sulfa drugs have increased risk of kernicterus in premature neonates. Tetracycline is avoided because of possibility of discoloration of teeth and hypoplasia of tooth enamel and long bone growth in the neonate. Also, the mother is at increased risk for acute fatty necrosis of the liver. Gentamicin is not indicated because of concern for possible ototoxicity in the neonate.

497. The answer is d. *(Braunwald, 15/e, pp 1360–1361.)* By definition, peripartum cardiomyopathy is cardiac dilatation and CHF of unexplained cause occurring during the last trimester of pregnancy or within 6 months of delivery. Half of patients will completely recover normal cardiac size and function. However, further pregnancies frequently produce increasing myocardial damage and increased mortality, and patients should be counseled to avoid future pregnancies. Treatment is the same as for other types of dilated cardiomyopathies and includes salt restriction, angiotensin converting enzyme inhibitors, diuretics, and digitalis and/or beta-blockers for symptomatic treatment. Other treatment modalities may include anticoagulation to prevent systemic embolization and an implantable cardioverter-defibrillator in patients with arrhythmias.

498. The answer is c. *(Gaster, pp 152–156.)* The patient is attempting to self-treat her depressive symptoms with St. John's wort, which has been reported to interact with certain prescription medications, including digoxin. St. John's wort may lower levels of digoxin by 25%. Another interaction that could be important in this case is bleeding, which has been reported in patients taking warfarin and Ginkgo biloba.

499. The answer is b. *(Carr, 1/e, p 149. Braunwald, 15/e, p 573.)* Palpable breast mass evaluation should determine whether the patient has a true mass or prominent physiologic glandular tissue. The next step is to determine if the dominant mass represents a cyst, benign solid mass, or cancer. The physical characteristics of this patient's mass that cause concern include irregular borders, size larger than 1 cm, and location in the upper outer quadrant of the breast. This patient's age (>35) also places her at slightly higher risk. Therefore repeat imaging including ultrasound is warranted. If no cyst is found and mammogram is negative, the patient should be examined by a breast surgeon or a comprehensive breast radiologist and biopsy performed. Six months is too long to reevaluate. In a younger woman (<35), repeat exam after the next menstrual cycle might be warranted (i.e., <1-month reevaluation). Assuming benign breast changes without further investigation is not appropriate. CT scanning does not currently provide useful information in the evaluation of palpable breast mass.

500. The answer is c. *(Braunwald, 15/e, p 1509.)* This patient's history and physical are consistent with a pulmonary embolus. The combination of respiratory distress, hypoxia, tachycardia, clear chest x-ray, and typical ECG changes makes this the most likely choice. There is no evidence on chest x-ray of infiltrate or metastatic disease. An anxiety attack would not cause hypoxia. Tamoxifen is associated with an increased risk of thromboembolic events.

Bibliography

Braunwald E, Fauci AS, Kasper DL, Hauser SL, et al (eds): *Harrison's Principles of Internal Medicine*, 15/e. New York, McGraw-Hill, 2001.

Braverman LE, Utiger RD (eds): *Werner & Ingbar's The Thyroid. A Fundamental and Clinical Text*, 8/e. New York, Lippincott Williams & Wilkins, 2000.

Carr PL, Freund KM, Somani S (eds): *Medical Care of Women*, 1/e. Philadelphia, Saunders, 1995.

Cummins RO (ed): *ACLS Provider Manual*, 1/e, Dallas, TX, American Heart Association, 2001.

Executive Summary of the Third Report of the National Cholesterol Education Program (NCEP) Expert Panel on Detection, Evaluation, and Treatment of High Blood Cholesterol in Adults (Adult Treatment Panel III). *JAMA* 285:2486–2497, 2001.

Freedberg IM, Eisen AZ, Wolf K (eds): *Fitzpatrick's Dermatology in General Medicine*, 5/e. New York, McGraw-Hill, 1999.

Fuster V, Alexander RW, O'Rourke RA, et al (eds): *Hurst's The Heart*, 10/e. New York, McGraw-Hill, 2001.

Gantz NM, Brown RB, Berk SL, et al (eds): *Manual of Clinical Problems in Infectious Disease*, 4/e. Boston, Little, Brown, 1999.

Gaster B, Holroyd J: St. John's Wort for depression. *Arch Int Med* 160: 152–156, 2000.

Gorbach SL, Bartlett JG, Blacklow NR (eds): *Infectious Diseases*, 2/e. Philadelphia, Saunders, 1998.

Hazzard WR, Blass JP, Ettinger WH et al (eds): *Principles of Geriatric Medicine and Gerontology*, 4/e, New York, McGraw-Hill, 1999.

Henderson DA: Smallpox. Clinical and epidemiologic features. www.cdc.gov/ncidod/eid, 2002.

Hurst JW: *Medicine for the Practicing Physician*, 4/e. Appleton and Lange, 1996.

Joint National Committee on Prevention, Detection, Evaluation, and Treatment of High Blood Pressure. The Sixth Report of the Joint National Committee on Prevention, Detection, Evaluation, and Treatment of High Blood Pressure (JNC VI). Bethesda, MD, National Institutes of Health, National Heart, Lung, and Blood Institute, NIH Publication 98-4080, 1997.

Kane RL, Ouslander JG, Abrass IB: Essentials of Clinical Geriatrics, 4/e. New York, McGraw-Hill, 1999.

Mandell GL, Bennett JE, Dolin R (eds): *Principles and Practice of Infectious Diseases*, 5/e. New York, Churchill Livingstone, 2000.

Physican's Desk Reference, 56/e. Montvale, NJ, Medical Economics, 2002.

Stein JH: *Internal Medicine*, 5/e. Boston, Little, Brown & Company, 1998.

Stobo JD, Hellman DB, Ladenson PW, et al (eds): *The Principles and Practice of Medicine*, 23/e. Stamford, CT, Appleton & Lange, 1996.

Index

A

Acetaminophen, 259, 263
Acromegaly, 111, 123
Actinomyces israelii, 5, 17
Acyclovir, 12, 24
Addison's disease, 108, 121–122, 176,
    190–191
Adenoma, prolactin-secreting, 106, 119
Adenosine, 76, 94
Adrenal tumor, 112, 124
Adult respiratory distress syndrome
    (ARDS), 15, 27, 58, 69
Advanced Cardiac Life Support (ACLS),
    77, 95
Agammaglobulinemia, 11, 23
AIDS (*see* HIV-positive patient)
Alcohol abuse, 234, 244
Allergy:
    food, 252, 256–257
    insect sting, 252, 257
Alpha blockers, 236, 244
Alzheimer's disease, 199, 208, 259,
    263–264
Amantadine, 6, 8, 18–19
Amaurosis fugax, 212
Amitriptyline, 34
Ampicillin, 11, 22
Amyotrophic lateral sclerosis (ALS), 37, 46,
    197, 205–206
Anaerobic infection, 48, 60
Anemia, 177, 179, 192
    hemolytic, 168, 175, 180, 190, 251
    microcytic, 167
Angina, 71, 90
Angiotensin converting enzyme (ACE)
    inhibitor, 73, 92, 155, 164, 236,
    244–245
Ankylosing spondylitis, 35, 40, 43
Anthrax, cutaneous, 221, 227
Antihistamines, 217, 224
Antineutrophil cytoplasmic antibodies
    (ANCA), 45
Antistreptolysin O antibody, 79, 96
Aortic regurgitation, 87, 99

Aortic stenosis, 74, 92, 234, 243
Aortoenteric fistula, 134, 144
Arrhenoblastoma, 114, 125
Arsenic poisoning, 237, 245
Arthritis, 259, 263
    acute septic, 39
    gout, 30, 39, 42, 236
    noninflammatory, 40
    rheumatoid, 29, 37–38, 46, 48, 57, 61,
    67
    (*See also* Felty syndrome; Polymyalgia
    rheumatica)
Ascites, 129, 139
Ascorbic acid, 217, 225
Aspergilloma, 18, 26
Aspergillus, 18, 253, 258
    A. flavus, 15
    A. fumigatus, 6–7, 18
Aspirin, 36, 44, 260
Asthma, 7, 18, 56–57, 66–67, 250
    hypertension and, 78, 95, 236, 245
    pulsus paradoxus and, 54, 64
Atheroembolic renal failure, 148, 158
Atrial contraction, premature (PAC), 75
Atrial fibrillation, 76, 93, 273
Atrial septal defect, 86, 99
Atrioventricular (AV) block, 71, 85, 90, 94,
    98
Atropine, 87, 100
A_1 antitrypsin deficiency, 57, 68

B

Back pain, 31, 40
Bacteremia, 12, 24
β-adrenergic agents, 100
    (*See also* Propanolol)
Barrett's esophagus, 140
Behçet syndrome, 35, 43
Bereavement support, 261, 265
Beta blockers, 230, 236, 240, 244–245
Biopsy, surgical, 178, 193, 219, 225, 274,
    279
Bisphosphonates, 107, 121
Bitemporal hemianopsia, 111, 123

Blastomycosis dermatitis, 6–7, 18
Blindness:
    sudden monocular, 203, 212
    transient, 196, 204
Body mass index (BMI), 270, 277
Bone densitometry, central, 275
Borrelia burgdorferi, 19
Brain abscess, 200, 209
Breast cancer, 233, 243, 274, 279–280
    diabetes and, 115, 126
    metastatic, 174, 189
Bronchiectasis, 57, 68
Bronchitis, 68, 249
Bronchospasm, 250, 255
Brown recluse spider, 237, 245

C
CAGE screening, 234, 244
Calcitonin, 107, 121
Calcium channel blocker, 87, 100
Calcium oxalate, 156, 165
Calcium pyrophosphate dihydrate deposition disease, 42
Candida albicans, 15, 26
Captopril, 88, 100
Carcinoma:
    hepatocellular, 173, 188
    metastatic, 174, 189
    renal, 171, 184
    small cell, 111, 124, 174, 189, 193
    (*See also specific type*)
Cardiac tamponade, 97
Cardiomyopathy:
    hypertrophic, 87, 99–100
    peripartum, 92, 273, 279
    postpartum, 73, 92
Carotid disease (*see* Cerebrovascular disease)
Carpal tunnel syndrome, 37, 46
Ceftriaxone, 8, 12, 14, 19, 24, 26
Cephalexin, 272, 278
Cerebellar ataxia, acute, 11, 22
Cerebrovascular disease, 203, 212–213
Chickenpox, 11, 13, 22–23, 25, 222, 228
Chlamydia trachomatis, 14, 24, 26
Chloramphenicol, 25
Chloroquine, 36, 44
Cholecystitis, 138

Cholesterol levels, 230–231, 241
Chronic obstructive pulmonary disease
    (COPD), 47, 52, 56, 62, 66–67
Ciprofloxacin, 235, 244
Cirrhosis, 63, 131, 141, 173, 188
Clostridium difficile, 134, 143
Coccidioides immitis, 15
Coccidioidomycosis, 27
Colitis, 134–135, 143–145
Complement deficiency C5–C9, 253, 257
Condyloma acuminatum, 18
Congestive heart failure, 48, 54, 56,
    61–63, 72–73, 91–92
    in geriatric patients, 261, 265
Contact dermatitis, 216, 223
Continuous positive airway pressure, 59,
    70
Coronary artery disease, 269, 276
Cor pulmonale, 84, 98
Corticosteroids, 4, 17, 79, 96
Coumadin (*see* Warfarin)
Coxsackievirus B, 15, 27
Creutzfeldt-Jakob disease, 199, 208
Crohn's disease, 135, 145
Cryoglobulinemia, essential mixed, 154,
    164
Cryptosporidium, 12, 23
Cushing's disease, 106, 119
Cystic fibrosis, 57, 68
Cystine, 156, 165
Cytomegalovirus, 12, 18, 23
C1 inhibitor deficiency, 251, 255

D
Danaparoid, 173, 187
Decay-accelerating factor deficiency, 251,
    255
Deep vein thrombosis (DVT), 65–66, 151
Defibrillation, 78, 95
Delirium, 199, 208
Dementia:
    Lewy body, 260, 263–264
    multi-infarct, 199, 208
    senile, 199, 208
Depression, 234, 244
De Quervain's disease, 37, 46, 117
Dermatomyositis, 209
Dexa scan, 268

Diabetes, 7, 18, 77, 90, 229, 236
  cholesterol levels in, 231, 241, 244
  coma and, 103, 116
  diet and, 104, 106, 117, 119–120
  exercise programs and, 106, 119
  in geriatric patients, 71, 148, 154, 163,
    237
  hypertension and, 155, 164, 229, 240
  impotence and, 107, 120
  insipidus, 115, 126
  mellitus, 67, 109, 115, 155, 173, 246
  pancreatitis and, 133, 143
Diabetic ketoacidosis (DKA), 18, 67
Dialysis, 148, 158
Diarrhea, 12, 23, 150, 160, 232
  antibiotic-induced, 134, 143–144
  chronic idiopathic, 249, 254
Digoxin, 81, 96, 261, 265, 273
Dilantin, 218, 225
Disseminated intravascular coagulation
    (DIC), 22, 191
Diuretics, 236, 245, 262, 266
Diverticulitis, 127–128, 132, 137–138, 141
Domestic abuse, 272, 278
Donepezil, 259, 263
Doxycycline, 12, 24–25
Dressler syndrome (*see* Post-cardiac injury
    syndrome)
Drug abuse, 235, 244
Drug screen, urine, 244
Dual x-ray absorptiometry, 268
Duodenal ulcer, 128, 132, 138
Dysentery, amebic, 145

E
Echocardiogram, 83, 97
Echovirus, 11, 23
Ectopic ACTH-producing neoplasm, 112,
    124
Edema, 72, 84, 151
Electromyography, 197
Emphysema, 58
Empty sella syndrome, 106, 119
Empyema, 48, 61
Encephalitis, 15, 26
Endocarditis:
  bacterial, subacute, 17
  infective, 22, 86, 98–99

Epiglottitis, acute, 1, 16
Epinephrine, 238, 246, 250, 255
Epstein-Barr virus, 11, 17, 22
Erysipelas, 26
Erythema infectiosum (*see* Fifth disease)
Erythema multiforme, 218, 225
Erythema nodosum, 217, 224
Erythromycin, 3
Escherichia coli, 9, 20
Esophageal cancer, 130, 140
Exercise programs, 106, 119, 261, 264

F
Fat embolism, 52, 62
Felty syndrome, 44
Fenfluramines, 69
Fever of unknown origin (FUO), 10,
    20–21
Fibromyalgia, 43, 46
Fifth disease, 15, 22, 27
Focal sclerosis, 156, 165
Focal segmental sclerosis, 152, 161
Framingham criteria, 72, 91

G
Gallstones, 137, 139
Ganciclovir, 6, 18
Gastric ulcer, 134, 144
Gastrinoma, 115, 125–126
Gastroesophageal reflux disease (GERD),
    140
Gastrointestinal bleeding, 36
Genital herpes, 12, 24
Gentamicin, 13, 24
Geriatric patients, 259–266
  exercise in, 261, 264
  medications to avoid in, 261, 265
Giant cell arteritis (*see* Temporal arteritis)
Giardia lamblia, 135, 145, 232, 242
Goldman index, 243
Gold therapy, 36, 44
Gonadotropin-releasing hormone (GnRH)
    analogue, 172, 187
Gonococcal infections, 12, 24
Goodpasture syndrome, 64
Gout (*See under* Arthritis)
Gram stain, 30, 51, 61
  sputum, 3, 8–9, 17, 19

Granulocytopenia, 36
Graves' disease, 105, 117–118, 123, 176,
    278
Guillain-Barré syndrome, 199, 207–208
G6PD deficiency, 132–133, 142

H
Haemophilus influenzae, 16
Hantavirus, 15, 27
Hashimoto's disease, 118
Headache, 195, 200, 202, 204, 209–211,
    236
Hearing loss, 262
Heart block, 80, 96
Helicobacter pylori, 128, 138–139
Hematocrit, 262, 266
Hematuria, 171, 185
Hemochromatosis, 173, 188
    arthropathy and, 33, 42, 114, 124, 132,
        142
Hemoptysis, 57, 68
Heparin, 71, 90, 187
Hepatic encephalopathy, 130, 140
Hepatitis, viral, 133, 143
Hepatitis B vaccine, 131, 141
Hepatoma, 173, 188
Herpes simplex type 2, 15, 26
Heterophile antibody test, 4, 17
Hip pain, 34, 43
Hives (*see* Urticaria)
HIV-positive patient, 149, 156, 165, 239,
    246–247
    immunizations for, 232, 242
    opportunistic infections in, 6, 12, 15,
        18, 23–24, 26
Hodgkin's disease, 172, 174, 186, 189,
    239, 247
Human papillomavirus (HPV), 18, 267,
    275
Humoral hypercalcemia of malignancy,
    177, 192
Huntingdon's chorea, 198, 207
Hydrocortisone, 109, 122
Hyperbilirubinemia, conjugated, 129, 139,
    142
Hyperglycemia, 103, 116–117
Hyperkalemia, 89, 101, 122, 154, 163
Hyperosmolar coma, 103, 116

Hypersensitivity pneumonitis, 47, 60, 252,
    256
Hypertension, 51, 62, 88, 108, 151, 161
    asthma and, 78, 95, 236, 245
    diabetes and, 155, 164, 229, 240
    diastolic, 121
    malignant, 95
    portal, 130, 139
    primary pulmonary, 59, 69
    refractory, 83, 97
    systolic, 266
Hyperthyroidism, surreptitious, 110, 123
Hypertriglyceridemia, 241
Hyperuricemia, asymptomatic, 238, 246
Hypocalcemia, 89, 101
Hypoglycemia:
    episodic, 109, 122
    factitious, 115, 126
    tumor-induced, 177, 192
Hypokalemia, 89, 101, 121
Hyponatremia, 89, 101, 122, 153, 162
    from inappropriate ADH secretion, 177,
        193
Hyporeninemic hypoaldosteronism, 154,
    163
Hypotension, postprandial, 261, 264–265
Hypothyroidism, 109, 118, 122
Hypoventilation, 67

I
IgA deficiency, 251, 256
IgE antibodies, 250, 254
IgM cold agglutinins, 3, 17
Imipenem, 13, 24
Immunodeficiency, common variable, 249,
    254
Impotence, 107, 120
Inappropriate antidiuretic hormone secre-
    tion, 123, 153, 162
Infectious mononucleosis, 17, 22
Influenza A, 6, 8, 18–19
Interferon α, 6, 18
Interferon β, 196, 205
Interleukin 12 receptor deficit, 253, 258
Intestinal obstruction, acute, 128, 138
Intrapulmonary hemorrhage, 54, 63
Intrinsic factor, 175, 190
Intubation, 52, 62

Irritable bowel syndrome, 133, 143
Isoniazid, 9, 239, 246–247
Isotretinoin, 215, 223

J
Jaundice, 129, 133, 139, 142

K
Koplik spots, 11, 23

L
Latex allergy, 250, 254–255
Lepirudin, 173, 187
Leukemia, chronic lymphocytic, 169, 182
Leukoplakia, 174, 188
Levodopa, 202, 211
Lewy body dementia, 260, 263
Lidocaine, 72, 91
Lipid profile, 267, 275
Lipomas, 178, 193
Liver abscess, 131–132, 141
Living will, 238, 245–246
Low-grade squamous intraepithelial lesion
    (LGSIL), 267
Loxosceles, 237, 245
Lung cancer, squamous cell, 170, 183
Lung scanning, 55, 65
Lyme disease, 7, 18–19
Lymphadenopathy, 172, 185–186
Lymphoreticular neoplasm, 251, 255

M
Malabsorption, 131, 141
Malaria, prophylaxis for, 175, 190
Malignant melanoma, 174, 189
Mallory-Weiss tear, 134, 144
Mammography, 233, 243
Measles, 11, 22–23, 220, 226
Medical nutrition therapy, 104, 117
Membranoproliferative glomerulonephritis,
    152, 162
Membranous nephropathy, 152, 161
Meningitis, 200, 209
Meningococcemia, 22, 257
Mesothelioma, 48, 61
Metabolic acidosis, anion-gap, 149, 159
Metabolic alkalosis, 151, 160–161
Methotrexate, 38

Metronidazole, 12, 24
Midbasilar artery disease, 212–213
Millard-Gubler syndrome, 210
Minimal change disease, 152, 161
Mitral stenosis, 74, 93
Mitral valve prolapse, 5, 10, 17, 21, 85, 98
Multiple cholesterol embolization syn-
    drome, 36, 45
Multiple endocrine neoplasia (MEN), 114,
    125
Multiple myeloma, 168–169, 180–181
Multiple sclerosis, 196, 204–205
Mumps, 11, 22
Myasthenia gravis, 13, 25, 197–198,
    206–207
Mycobacteria, 253, 258
Mycoplasma pneumoniae, 17, 168, 180
Myocardial infarction (MI), 71–73, 90, 92
    acute, 80, 82, 96, 260, 263
Myxedema coma, 122

N
Neisseria, 257
    N. gonorrhoeae, antibiotic-resistant, 24
    N. meningitidis, 11
Nephrectomy, 171, 184
Neutropenia, 253, 258
Nitroprusside, 78, 95
Non-anion-gap metabolic acidosis, 150,
    160
Nonsteroidal anti-inflammatory drug
    (NSAID), 72, 91

O
Obstructive sleep apnea syndrome, 70
Optic neuritis, 204
Osteoporosis, 36, 268, 275–276
Otitis externa, 1, 16
Ovarian cancer, 170, 183–184

P
Pacemaker, 80, 96
Paget's disease of bone, 107, 120–121
Pancreatic cancer, 132–133, 139, 142
Pancreatitis, 11, 22, 241
    acute, 127, 137, 231
    chronic, 133, 143
Pancytopenia, 183

Panic disorder, 231, 241
Pap smear, 267
Paraneoplastic syndrome, 177, 192
Parkinson's disease (PD), 198, 202, 207,
    211, 220, 264
Parvovirus B19, 11, 15, 22, 27
Patient autonomy, 237–238, 245
Penicillin, 2, 8, 12, 16, 19, 24, 65, 79, 96
Peptic ulcer disease, 115, 125, 138
Pericarditis, 97, 231, 242
Peripheral vascular disease, 237
Pernicious anemia, 175, 190
Petechiae, 11, 22
Pheochromocytoma, 110, 123, 125
Photosensitivity, 13, 24
Pituitary tumor, 112, 124
Pityriasis rosea, 220, 226
Plasma osmolality, 150, 159
Pleural effusion, 47–48, 54, 60, 63
Pneumocystis carnii, 12, 23, 25
Pneumonia, 12, 62, 67
    with adult respiratory distress syn-
        drome, 15
    community-acquired, 19, 64
    hypersensitivity pneumonitis, 60, 252,
        256
    M. pneumoniae (see Mycoplasma
        pneumoniae)
    pneumococcal, 65
    S. pneumoniae (see Streptococcus
        pneumoniae)
    varicella, 25
    (See also specific pathogen)
Pneumonia vaccine, 262, 266
Pneumothorax, 58, 68–69
Poison ivy, 221, 227
Polyarteritis nodosa, 35–36, 43, 45, 154,
    163
Polymyalgia rheumatica, 35, 42, 44
Polymyositis, 201, 209–210
Polysomnography, 59, 70
Post-cardiac injury syndrome, 91
Prednisone, 25, 36, 44
Pregnancy, 237, 245
Presbycusis, 262, 266
Prolactinoma, 106, 119
Propanolol, 87–88, 100

Propionibacterium acnes, 223
Propylthiouracil, 176, 191
Prostate cancer, 172, 186–187
Prostatic hypertrophy, benign, 236
Proteinuria, 36
Providencia stuartii, 5
Pseudogout, 42
Pseudomonas aeruginosa, 1, 16, 57, 68
Psoriasis, 215, 223
Pulmonary embolism, 56, 65–67, 91,
    274
Pulmonary hypertension, primary, 59, 69
Pulmonary vasodilator, acute drug testing
    with, 59, 69
Pulsus paradoxus, 54, 64, 83, 97

R
Rabies, 10, 21
Radiocontrast media sensitivity, 250, 255
Ranitidine, 130
Raynaud's phenomenon, 32, 41
Reiter syndrome, 32, 41
Renal failure, acute (ARF), rhabdomyolysis-
    induced, 147–148, 157–158
Renin-angiotensin-aldosterone system,
    defects in, 154, 163
Respiratory acidosis, acute, 67
Respiratory alkalosis, acute, 67
Respiratory syncytial virus (RSV), 6, 18
Restraints, use of, 260, 264
Retinitis, 12, 23
Retinopathy, 36
Rhabdomyolysis-induced acute renal
    failure (ARF), 147–148, 157–158
Rheumatic fever, 74, 93, 95–96
Ribavirin, 6, 18
Rickettsial disease, 22, 25
Rifampin, 9
Riluzole, 197, 206
Rocky Mountain spotted fever, 14, 25,
    216, 223
Rosacea, 221, 227
Rubeola (see Measles)

S
Salmonella, 12, 24, 41, 146
Sarcoidosis, 53, 57, 62, 68

Sarcoma, soft tissue, 193
Scleroderma, 32, 41
Sclerosing cholangitis, 131–132, 142
Scrotum, mass in, 171, 184–185
Scurvy, 217, 224
Seborrheic dermatitis, 220, 226
Second heart sound (S₂), paradoxical splitting of, 86, 99
Seizures, 12, 24, 153, 162
    absence, 202, 211–212
    atonic, 202, 212
    complex partial, 202, 212
    simple partial, 212
Sepsis, 22, 58, 69
    post-splenectomy, 253, 258
Serum osmolarity, 103, 116
Shigella, 41
    S. dysenteriae, 135, 145–146
Sickle cell anemia, 5, 9, 18, 175, 190
Silver methenamine stain, 13, 25
Sinus bradycardia, 100
Sjögren syndrome, 30, 38
Skin, desquamation of, 11, 22
Smallpox, 11, 23, 222, 228
Smokers, tobacco, 170, 174, 183, 233, 267, 275
Smoking cessation programs, 58, 68
Spironolactone, 88, 100
Splenomegaly, 175, 190
Sprue, 141
St. John's wort, 273, 279
Staphylococci, methicillin-resistant, 8, 19
Staphylococcus aureus, 11, 22, 30, 39, 61–62, 135, 145
Statin drugs, 230, 240
Stomatitis, 36, 44
Streptococcus pneumoniae, 19, 55, 64, 180, 253, 258
    sickle cell anemia and, 5, 9, 18
Streptococcus pyogenes, 14, 26
Stress test, 269, 277
Struvite, 156, 165
Syncope, 195, 204, 261
Syphilis, 12, 16, 24
Systemic lupus erythematosus (SLE), 32, 40–41, 154, 164

T
Tachycardia, supraventricular, 76, 94
Tachypnea, 56, 66
Takayasu's arteritis, 36, 45
Tamoxifen, 274, 280
Telangiectasia, hereditary hemorrhagic (HHT), 134, 144
Temporal arteritis, 33, 42, 45, 200, 209
Terazosin, 88, 100
Testicular cancer, 174, 185, 189
Tetanus-diphtheria toxoid booster, 232, 242, 262, 266
Tetracycline, 13, 24
Thallium scanning, 269, 277
Thermophilic actinomycetes, 252, 256
Thrombocytopenia, drug-induced, 173, 187
Thrombophlebitis, 173, 177, 192
Thymoma, 198, 207
Thyroid, medullary carcinoma of, 114, 125
Thyroiditis, 105, 110, 117–118, 123
    postpartum, 271–272, 277–278
Thyroid nodule, 105, 118
Thyroid peroxidase antibody (TPO), 105, 118
Thyrotoxicosis, 104–105, 117, 277
Ticks, 14, 25
Tinea versicolor, 220, 227
Toxoplasma gondii, 12
Toxoplasmosis, 24
Transient ischemic attack (TIA), 173
Trichomoniasis, 12, 24
Tricuspid regurgitation, 87, 99
Trimethoprim-sulfamethoxazole, 14, 25, 149, 158
Tuberculosis, 15, 26, 48, 61–62
    Addison's disease and, 108–109, 121–122
    isoniazid prophylaxis for, 239, 246–247
    multidrug-resistant, 9, 20
Tubular necrosis, acute, 13, 24

U
Ulcer, gastrointestinal (*see specific type*)
Upper respiratory infection, 17
Urethritis, 12, 24

Uric acid, 156, 165
Urinary tract infection (UTI), 272, 278
Urticaria, 216–217, 224, 249, 254

V
Vaccininea necrosum, 222, 228
Vancomycin, 19
Varicella (*see* Chickenpox)
Venereal Disease Research Laboratory
(VDRL) est, 2
Venereal warts, 6, 18
Ventricular contraction, premature (PVC),
75, 93
Ventricular fibrillation, 95
Ventricular septal defect, 75, 93
Ventricular tachycardia, 72, 78, 95
Viridans streptococci, 5, 17
Vitamin B_{12} deficiency, 169, 175, 181–182,
190

W
Warfarin, 76, 93–94
drug interactions with, 173, 188, 235,
244, 273, 279
pulmonary embolus and, 56, 66, 235
Wegener's granulomatosis, 36, 45, 154,
164
Wenckebach phenomenon, 77, 94
Wilson's disease, 114, 124, 198, 207
Wiskott-Aldrich syndrome, 251, 255

X
Xanthoma, 219, 225
X-ray, chest, 233, 242
XXY karyotype, 113, 124

Z
Zollinger-Ellison syndrome, 132, 142
Zygomycosis, 6–7, 18